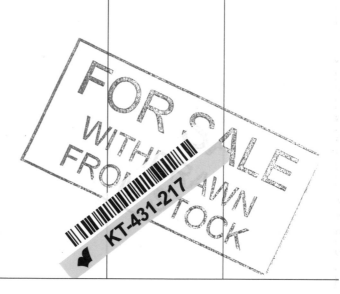

Overcoming Common Problems Series

Selected titles

A full list of titles is available from Sheldon Press,
36 Causton Street, London SW1P 4ST and on our website at
www.sheldonpress.co.uk

Breast Cancer: Your treatment choices
Dr Terry Priestman

Chronic Fatigue Syndrome: What you need to know about CFS/ME
Dr Megan A. Arroll

Cider Vinegar
Margaret Hills

Coeliac Disease: What you need to know
Alex Gazzola

Coping Successfully with Hiatus Hernia
Dr Tom Smith

Coping with Difficult Families
Dr Jane McGregor and Tim McGregor

Coping with Epilepsy
Dr Pamela Crawford and Fiona Marshall

Coping with Memory Problems
Dr Sallie Baxendale

Coping with the Psychological Effects of Illness
Dr Fran Smith, Dr Carina Eriksen
and Professor Robert Bor

Coping with Schizophrenia
Professor Kevin Gournay and Debbie Robson

Coping with Thyroid Disease
Mark Greener

Depressive Illness: The curse of the strong
Dr Tim Cantopher

Dr Dawn's Guide to Brain Health
Dr Dawn Harper

Dr Dawn's Guide to Heart Health
Dr Dawn Harper

Dr Dawn's Guide to Weight and Diabetes
Dr Dawn Harper

Dr Dawn's Guide to Women's Health
Dr Dawn Harper

The Empathy Trap: Understanding antisocial personalities
Dr Jane McGregor and Tim McGregor

The Fibromyalgia Healing Diet
Christine Craggs-Hinton

Fibromyalgia: Your treatment guide
Christine Craggs-Hinton

Helping Elderly Relatives
Jill Eckersley

The Holistic Health Handbook
Mark Greener

How to Stop Worrying
Dr Frank Tallis

Invisible Illness: Coping with misunderstood conditions
Dr Megan A. Arroll and Professor
Christine P. Dancey

Living with the Challenges of Dementia: A guide for family and friends
Patrick McCurry

Living with Complicated Grief
Professor Craig A. White

Living with Fibromyalgia
Christine Craggs-Hinton

Living with Hearing Loss
Dr Don McFerran, Lucy Handscomb
and Dr Cherilee Rutherford

Overcoming Fear with Mindfulness
Deborah Ward

Overcoming Low Self-esteem with Mindfulness
Deborah Ward

Overcoming Stress
Professor Robert Bor, Dr Carina Eriksen
and Dr Sara Chaudry

Overcoming Worry and Anxiety
Dr Jerry Kennard

Physical Intelligence: How to take charge of your weight
Dr Tom Smith

Post-Traumatic Stress Disorder: Recovery after accident and disaster
Professor Kevin Gournay

The Self-Esteem Journal
Alison Waines

The Stroke Survival Guide
Mark Greener

Ten Steps to Positive Living
Dr Windy Dryden

Treating Arthritis: The drug-free way
Margaret Hills and Christine Horner

Understanding High Blood Pressure
Dr Shahid Aziz and Dr Zara Aziz

Understanding Yourself and Others: Practical ideas from the world of coaching
Bob Thomson

When Someone You Love Has Depression: A handbook for family and friends
Barbara Baker

Overcoming Common Problems

Dr Dawn's Guide to Brain Health

DR DAWN HARPER

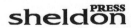

First published in Great Britain in 2015

Sheldon Press
36 Causton Street
London SW1P 4ST
www.sheldonpress.co.uk

British Library Cataloguing-in-Publication Data
A catalogue record for this book is available from the British Library

ISBN 978–1–84709–360–8
eBook ISBN 978–1–84709–361–5

Typeset by Fakenham Prepress Solutions, Fakenham, Norfolk NR21 8NN
First printed in Great Britain by Ashford Colour Press
Subsequently digitally reprinted in Great Britain

eBook by Fakenham Prepress Solutions, Fakenham, Norfolk NR21 8NN

Produced on paper from sustainable forests

Dedicated to my three beautiful children
Charlie, Eleanor and Harvey

Contents

Note to the reader

This is not a medical book and is not intended to replace advice from your doctor. Consult your pharmacist or doctor if you believe you have any of the symptoms described, and if you think you might need medical help.

1

The nervous system

Everything we do, think or feel is controlled by our brain and nervous system. We have over 100,000 million nerve cells, each one with around 10,000 connections, which makes us the most complicated machines in the world. Our nervous system can be thought of as having three parts:

- the central nervous system, made up of the brain and spinal cord;
- the peripheral nervous system, the nerves that supply all the different parts of the body;
- the autonomic nervous system, which controls automatic functions such as breathing and heart rate.

The average brain weighs around 1.4 kg. Its surface is covered by a thin layer called the **cerebral cortex**, which is a mass of ridges and furrows. If spread out flat, it would cover an area of one square metre!

The central nervous system

The brain

The **cerebrum** is the largest part of the brain, also referred to as the **forebrain**. It is divided into two halves called the **left and right cerebral hemispheres**. The right hemisphere controls the left side of the body and the left hemisphere controls the right side of the body. Each cerebral hemisphere is divided into lobes.

- The frontal lobe is responsible for speech, personality, problem solving, movement and sensation.

- The temporal lobe is responsible for processing sound and storing memory.
- The parietal lobe is responsible for touch, temperature, pressure, pain and processing speech.
- The occipital lobe is responsible for vision.

The **brain stem** connects the cerebrum and cerebellum to the spinal cord and is responsible for all essential functions of life, such as breathing and heart rate. The **cerebellum** is also sometimes called the **hindbrain** and is responsible for balance, posture and co-ordination. The **pituitary gland** produces hormones that control growth, metabolism, menstruation, fertility and breast milk production. The **pineal gland** produces melatonin and controls sleep.

The brain is covered by three layers of membranes, called the **meninges**, which also cover the spinal cord. The meninges are the:

- **dura mater**, the tough outer protective layer;
- **arachnoid mater**, the middle layer;
- **pia mater**, the delicate inner layer.

The spinal cord

The spinal cord is like an electrical motorway relaying messages to and from the brain and the rest of the body. It consists of 31 pairs of spinal nerves, which provide a two-way communication system between the spinal cord and the rest of the body. Unlike the cranial nerves, they don't have specific names but are referred to according to the level at which they leave the spinal cord. There are eight pairs of cervical nerves, twelve pairs of thoracic nerves, five pairs of lumbar nerves, five pairs of sacral nerves and one pair of coccygeal nerves.

The space surrounding the organs of the central nervous system is filled with a clear fluid called the cerebrospinal fluid (CSF), which protects the brain and spinal cord, supplies nutrients to the tissues and removes waste products of metabolism.

The peripheral nervous system

The peripheral nervous system refers to all the parts of the nervous system outside the brain and spinal cord and includes the cranial nerves, motor nerves and sensory nerves.

The cranial nerves

There are 12 cranial nerves that emerge from the base of the brain.

1 The olfactory nerve is responsible for the sense of smell.
2 The optic nerve is responsible for vision.
3 The oculomotor nerve is responsible for eye movements and focus.
4 The trochlear nerve is also responsible for eye movements and focus.
5 The trigeminal nerve is responsible for sensation in the face and the muscles of chewing.
6 The abducens nerve is responsible for eye movements and focus.
7 The facial nerve is responsible for facial movements and taste.
8 The vestibulocochlear nerve is responsible for balance and hearing.
9 The glossopharyngeal nerve is responsible for swallowing and taste at the back of the tongue.
10 The vagus nerve is responsible for the gag reflex, and vocal cord movement.
11 The accessory nerve is responsible for head movements and shoulder shrugging.
12 The hypoglossal nerve is responsible for tongue movement and swallowing.

The motor nerves

Motor nerves (or neurons) carry signals from the brain and spinal cord to the rest of your body to tell your muscles to contract. They have a cell body at the end closest to the central nervous system, with a long stem called an axon and lots of finger-like projections at the other end called dendrites.

The sensory nerves

Sensory nerves are responsible for relaying information from the rest of your body back to the brain and spinal cord. There are different types of sensory nerves that are responsible for pain, temperature, touch and joint position sense. Unlike motor neurons, they have dendrites at both ends, connected by a long axon and a cell body in the middle.

The interneurons

These neurons connect the motor and sensory pathways. The axons of the nerves are covered in a protective sheath called myelin, which increases the speed of nerve conduction.

The autonomic nervous system

This is the part of the nervous system that continues to work automatically without any conscious awareness on our part. It is responsible for heart rate, breathing, temperature control and digestion. It can be thought of in two parts: the sympathetic and parasympathetic nervous systems.

The sympathetic nervous system

The sympathetic nervous system provides the 'fight or flight' mechanism. When triggered, during times of stress, exercise or emotion, it causes your heart rate to increase, your breathing to quicken and digestion to slow to allow blood to be diverted to the muscles of the limbs should you need to run away from danger.

The parasympathetic nervous system

The parasympathetic nervous system is the opposite to the sympathetic system and works to undo the effects of 'fight or flight'. It slows heart rate and respiration and increases digestion.

Examination of the nervous system

You may not realize it but your doctor will begin his examination of your nervous system the moment you walk through the door. He or she will note the way you walk, whether you have a limp or whether you drag a foot. Your doctor will note if there is any asymmetry to your face and whether you have a tremor. As soon as you speak, your doctor will notice if you have any slurring to your speech or if your voice is hoarse. Doctors rarely do a full neurological assessment, outside of an exam setting, but will take a detailed medical history and then hone in on the relevant parts of the examination, as I will describe in this chapter.

Examination of the cranial nerves

Olfactory nerve Your doctor will ask you to close each nostril in turn and ask you to identify the smell in different bottles that usually contain easily recognizable odours such as peppermint, vanilla and coffee.

Optic nerve Your doctor will start by testing your visual acuity (your ability to see). To do this he or she will use a chart of letters called a Snellen chart and you will be asked to stand a set distance from the chart and read out the letters as far down the chart as you can. Each eye is tested separately by covering the other eye. If you wear glasses you will be allowed to keep them on during this test. You will then be asked to sit opposite your doctor and stare into your doctor's eyes. Your doctor will extend his arm and point in four directions – as far as he or she can reach up and to the right, up and to the left, down and to the right, and down and to the left. He or she will then start to bring his or her finger in toward the centre and will ask you to tell him when his or her finger is in vision. This tells him how your visual fields compare to your doctor's. Your doctor will ask you to cover one eye and he or she will cover one eye and then will gradually move a pin, with a round, red head, horizontally across your field of vision to compare your blind spot with his or her blind spot. We all have a blind spot where, momentarily, we will not be able to see the pin. He or she will then shine a light in each eye to check that the pupil reacts appropriately. Finally, your doctor will use an ophthalmoscope to look at the back of the eye to check that the optic disc (the place where the optic nerve comes into the back of the eye) is healthy.

Oculomotor, trochlear and abducens nerves These nerves control eye movements. To check that they are all working properly, your doctor will ask you to sit in front of him or her and follow his or her finger with your eyes, keeping your head absolutely still. He or she will move the finger around to check that your eyes can move in all directions and symmetrically. He or she will then move the finger toward your nose, which should make you go cross-eyed.

Trigeminal nerve Your doctor will lightly brush your forehead, cheek and chin on each side of your face to test sensation. He or she will want to know if it feels normal and if all areas feel the same. Your doctor will then ask you to clench your teeth to check that the muscles used for chewing are strong. He or she will take a small spindle of cotton wool and gently touch the outside of the whites of your eyes. This should make you blink. It is called the corneal reflex.

Facial nerve Your doctor will ask you to smile, testing for symmetry. He or she will ask you to screw your eyes tightly shut and will try to gently open them and will then ask you to raise your eyebrows.

Glossopharyngeal and vagus nerves Your doctor will ask you to open you mouth and say 'Ahh'. This is checking for a normal sound, and he or she will also look at the uvula, the piece of tissue hanging down at the back of the roof of your mouth, to check that it is in the midline. He or she will then test your gag reflex by touching the back of the tongue and ask you to puff out your cheeks to check that the muscles supplied by these nerves are all responding correctly.

Accessory nerve Your doctor will ask you to shrug your shoulders and keep them up while he or she pushes down; he or she will ask you to turn your head to each side and resist while your doctor tries to turn it back.

Hypoglossal nerve Your doctor will ask you to stick out your tongue. He or she will check that it is straight and not deviating to one side.

Examination of the sensory system

Sensory fibres supply sensation to the skin in bands, known as **dermatomes**, and your doctor will want to check any dermatomes he or she suspects may be causing problems. Your doctor will test the four modalities of sensation.

- *Light touch and pinprick* Your doctor will use his or her finger, or a cotton wool ball, to lightly touch your skin and a pin, such as one that is used to check blood glucose, which is then disposed of after use. He or she will want to know that these sensations feel normal and, also, that they are the same in different parts of your body.
- *Proprioception (joint position sense)* Your doctor will ask you to close your eyes and will hold the sides of your big toe or one of your fingers. He or she will bend the joint down, and tell you that is down, and up, and tell you that is up. He or she will then move the joint up and down randomly and ask you which way the joint is moving.
- *Temperature* Your doctor will use a metal tuning fork, for

example, to see if you can feel a cold sensation on your skin.

- *Vibration sense* He or she will then prime the tuning fork and place the base on your skin to check that you can feel the vibrations.

Examination of the motor system

The examination of the motor system started as you walked through the door, but when your doctor has got you on the examination couch, he or she will start by looking at your muscles to see if there is any wasting. He or she will also look for tiny involuntary movements, and will then look at four different modalities of the motor system.

- *Tone* Your doctor will pick up your limbs one by one, and ask you to relax completely to check the tone of the muscles. He or she may flex your elbow, asking you to remain totally floppy and rotate your wrist, looking for evidence of cogwheel rigidity as seen in Parkinson's disease. He or she may force your ankle into flexion by pressing on the ball of your foot to bring your toes up toward your shin. If the foot quivers, this suggests increased tone.
- *Power* Your doctor will test the power of various muscles by asking you to maintain a specific position and resist him or her trying to move you out of it. Power is graded between 0 and 5, where 0 is no movement in a muscle at all and 5 is normal power.
- *Reflexes* Your doctor will use a tendon hammer to try to elicit reflexes by tapping in the crease of your elbow and below your patella. If your doctor cannot elicit a reflex, he or she may ask you to lock your fingers and pull against yourself while clenching your teeth, as this can make the reflex more prominent. Your doctor will use the other end of the hammer to stroke the sole of your foot to see if your big toe moves in a reflex reaction.
- *Co-ordination* Your doctor may ask you to tap the back of

your hand with the other hand and then rapidly twist the tapping hand back and fore. Your doctor will then ask you to swap sides. He or she will ask you to touch his or her finger, which will be at the full stretch of your reach, and then touch the tip of your nose. Your doctor will move his or her finger around and ask you to keep alternating finger and nose as fast as you can. He or she will do this with both hands to check co-ordination. Your doctor may then ask you to walk a straight line, placing your heel immediately in front of your toes. Finally, he or she will ask you to stand with your feet together and to close your eyes, to check that you can maintain your balance.

Tests on the nervous system

After taking a history from you about your symptoms and examining you, your doctor will have what we call a differential diagnosis in his head. I was once told, by a very wise professor, that a good doctor spends most of his time listening. By the time he or she has finished listening, he or she will know what examination he or she needs to perform to rule out or rule in certain possibilities and by the time he or she has finished examining, he or she should know what tests are necessary to confirm the working diagnosis. Below are some of the diagnostic tests used to check your nervous system:

Skull X-rays These are used to look for fractures. They can also show if there are cancerous deposits called **metastases**.

Spinal X-rays These will show fractures, congenital malformations, infection (**osteomyelitis**) and metastases.

CT scan A CT (**computed tomography**) scan is used to look for tumours, bleeding and excess fluid, but it has its limitations. It is not good at looking at the base of the brain and it is not sensitive enough to pick up lesions, such as plaques of multiple sclerosis and some blood clots.

MRI scan An MRI (**magnetic resonance imaging**) scan gives a more detailed picture than a CT scan. It shows individual nerves and is much better at detecting problems in the base of the brain, plaques of multiple sclerosis, tumours, bleeds and tissue death. It uses magnets, rather than radiation, to produce the scan, which means that patients with metalwork in their bodies, such as pacemakers for example, cannot have an MRI. There are specialized MRI scans and these include:

• *Functional MRI* During this type of scan you will be asked to do certain things, such as move your arm or read something, so that the doctors can look at the way your brain reacts in specific circumstances.
• *MR angiography* This looks at the blood vessels in detail.
• *MR spectroscopy* This looks at the chemicals in a known tumour.

PET scan A PET (**positron emission tomography**) scan involves having an injection of a small amount of a radioactive substance; this is taken up by the brain and the PET scan measures how quickly this happens in different areas and can be useful in working out whether a tumour is cancerous or not.

SPECT scan A SPECT (**single photon emission computed tomography**) scan is similar to a PET scan in that you will have an injection of radioactive chemical, which is taken up by tumours.

EEG An EEG (**electroencephalogram**) involves having multiple electrodes attached to the scalp to monitor brain waves. It is particularly useful in diagnosing epilepsy as there are characteristic changes in the wave patterns in people who suffer with epilepsy.

VEP A VEP (**visually evoked potentials**) records the time it takes for a visual image to reach the brain. It used to be done to diagnose multiple sclerosis but it is used less frequently now that MRI scanning is more routinely available.

Lumbar puncture Lumbar puncture involves inserting a needle into the lumbar spine to remove some CSF. This is done most often to look for infections, such as meningitis or encephalitis, but it can also be done to check for the presence of blood in a suspected subarachnoid haemorrhage. The patient is asked to lie on the edge of the bed with their knees curled up and their chin on their chest. This position opens up the space between the vertebrae. The space between the third and fourth lumbar vertebra is marked. The skin is then cleaned and local anaesthetic is injected into the area. The lumbar puncture needle is pushed through the skin into the subdural space and the CSF pressure is measured before samples are collected and sent to the laboratory for analysis. The patient is asked to lie still for a while after the procedure to reduce the risk of developing a post-lumbar puncture headache.

Biopsy A biopsy is done under CT or MRI control to remove a sample of tissue. The tissue is analysed under a microscope, usually to assess the type of tumour.

Angiogram An angiogram is sometimes done to assess which blood vessels are supplying a tumour, or to see whether a tumour is attached to a collection of blood vessels, before deciding on possible surgery.

Myelogram A myelogram involves doing a lumbar puncture and injecting dye in the CSF and taking X-rays. This technique is used if it is suspected that a tumour is blocking the CSF and the individual cannot have an MRI scan.

Neuroendoscopy A neuroendoscopy is done under general anaesthetic and involves drilling a small hole in the skull, and then passing a telescope through to look directly at the brain. This is sometimes done to physically look for a suspected brain tumour.

2
Stroke and other cerebrovascular diseases

Cerebrovascular diseases are conditions that develop because of problems with the blood supply to the brain. There are four main types:

- stroke
- transient ischaemic attack
- subarachnoid haemorrhage
- multi-infarct (vascular) dementia.

In this chapter, I will discuss stroke and transient ischaemic attack. Subarachnoid haemorrhage is discussed in Chapter 3 and multi-infarct (vascular) dementia in Chapter 7.

Stroke

A stroke occurs when the blood supply to the brain is cut off. In eight out of ten cases this is due to a blood clot, which forms in an area of narrowed artery usually due to atherosclerosis. Our arteries harden as we age, but there are several lifestyle factors, which I will discuss in this chapter, that can speed up that process and, conversely, if we address those factors and alter our lifestyle we can reduce our risk. Given that there are over 150,000 strokes every year in the UK and that stroke is the commonest cause of adult disability worldwide, this is something we should take very seriously. My own late grandmother suffered a stroke and it was so sad to see such a vibrant woman become so incapacitated and dependent on others.

What causes a stroke?

In eight out of ten cases a stroke is caused by a blood clot but sometimes it may be caused by a bleed in the brain or, rarely, by inflammation in the blood vessels supplying the brain. The way we treat a stroke varies depending on the cause and the treatment is more effective the sooner it is given, so it is vital that if you suspect a stroke you call for urgent medical help.

How would I recognize a stroke?

Some of you may have seen the television adverts that explain what to look out for in someone having a stroke. These signs are summarised using the acronym FAST to help you remember:

- Face, there is an asymmetry of the face meaning that the person may be unable to smile on one side or has a droopy eye;
- Arm, the person may not be able to lift one arm;
- Speech may be slurred, the person may be talking gibberish or may not be able to talk at all;
- Time is of the essence. If you suspect a stroke, the sooner you can get medical help, the better the outlook. If you think this is happening to someone, call 999 immediately.

What happens after I call 999?

If a stroke is suspected, the medical team will order an urgent scan to assess whether the stroke has been caused by a bleed or a clot. If a clot is found, clot-busting drugs can be given; the more quickly these are given the more quickly the clot can be dispelled and blood supply restored to the brain. Every minute counts when dealing with a stroke so, if a clot is detected, the medical team will work hard to start this therapy as soon as possible. If you are not eligible for clot-busting drugs, you may be given aspirin or other drugs to make your blood less sticky, and if your doctors notice that your heart has an abnormal rhythm, called

atrial fibrillation, you will be given treatment for that to reduce your risk of further episodes. Once you have been stabilised, you will start on your rehabilitation, which is likely to involve lots of different people including physiotherapists, speech therapists, occupational therapists, psychologists and, of course, the doctors and nurses looking after you.

What are the long-term effects of a stroke?

About half of all stroke sufferers will be living independently six months after the event. Sadly, between 20 and 25 per cent of people who have a stroke will die as a result. Some make a full recovery although the rehabilitation may take months but others go on to have long-term disabilities, including:

- speech difficulties
- weakness
- co-ordination and balance problems
- difficulties swallowing
- emotional lability and depression
- problems with concentration
- visual problems
- fatigue.

The speech difficulties associated with stroke may result in people having difficulty expressing themselves. The person who has had the stroke may know what they want to say but use the wrong word. They may, for example, want to know where the keys are but ask for the car. Other stroke sufferers may not be able to understand you when you talk to them because the part of the brain that processes and understands speech has been damaged, and some will be unable to speak at all. The weakness can range from a total inability to move one side of the body to varying degrees of weakness in an arm and/or leg. The visual problems mean that sometimes people will have lost the ability to see anything on one side of their visual field.

What can I do to reduce my risks of having a stroke?

There are several changes to lifestyle that can influence your blood pressure and cholesterol level and could prevent you having a stroke.

- *Smoking* If you are a smoker you should stop now. Smoking doesn't necessarily cause a stroke but it adds to your risk. Your GP and pharmacist will be able to help you. Most surgeries now run smoking cessation clinics where you will be able to discuss which methods appeal most to you. Some people use nicotine replacement, others may choose pills to help with the cravings and some may swap to electronic vaping devices.
- *Weight* If you are overweight, you should aim to lose weight gradually – one to two pounds a week – until you are a healthy body mass index (BMI), which is between 18.5 and 25. Even small weight loss can make a big difference – just a one kilogram loss can equate to a fall in blood pressure of 1 mmHg and, if you are obese, a 10 per cent drop in body weight will equate to a 10 per cent drop in cholesterol. You can calculate your BMI by dividing your weight in kilos by the square of your height in metres. So, if I am 1.63 m tall and weigh 52 kg, my BMI is:

$$BMI = 52/ (1.63 \times 1.63) = 19.5$$

- *Diet* It is important that you aim to have a healthy well-balanced diet. Watch your fat intake – only a third of your total calories should be fat and you should limit your intake of trans fats and saturated fats to a third of your total fat intake. This means limiting your intake of butter, cheese, pastries, cakes and biscuits. It will also mean getting into the habit of checking food labels for fat content. This may seem laborious at first but you will soon get to know which foods you should avoid. You should eat at least five portions of fruit and vegetables a day. A portion is a single apple, orange or banana; two plums or apricots; 30 g of dried fruit; two broccoli spears; one medium tomato or seven cherry tomatoes; three heaped tablespoons of beans; or 150 ml of unsweetened fruit juice. However, because fruit juice has less fibre you can only count one glass into your five a day. And potatoes don't count as vegetables in this context. Watch your sugar intake too, and beware 'low fat' options – always check the labels as 'low fat' often means 'high sugar'. You should also eat two portions of oily fish each week; this includes mackerel, sardines, kippers, salmon, pilchards, herring or fresh tuna.

- *Salt* We have got used to a high salt diet in the western world. You should limit your daily intake to 6 g. Start by not adding salt to your food. At first this will taste bland but human taste buds adapt very quickly and by using herbs and spices you will soon wonder how you ever managed to eat such salty food! When you start looking at the hidden salt in processed foods you will be shocked by the amounts.

- *Exercise* You should aim to do half an hour of exercise at least five times a week. It doesn't matter what you do. It doesn't have to be in a fancy gym but you should choose something you enjoy doing so that you will stick with it and, even better, if you can exercise with a friend then you will encourage each other when your willpower is weak. So whether it's a brisk walk, cycling, jogging, swimming or dancing, you need to be exercising at a level that makes you out of breath. If you are gasping for breath then you should ease back a bit but if you can chat away easily while you are doing your exercise then you are kidding yourself and you need to up your game!

- *Alcohol* Drinking to excess can lead to an increase in blood pressure, which increases your risk of a stroke, so make sure you stick to recommended limits of alcohol – that is 14 units per week for women and 21 for men – and try to have at least two dry days per week. A unit is actually probably a lot less than you think. The simple way to calculate your alcohol intake is by looking at the percentage alcohol in the drink you are drinking. The percentage alcohol shows you the number of units in a litre of that drink; so, for wine, a 75 cl bottle is three-quarters of a litre (75 cl = 750 ml; 1 litre = 1000 ml), so if the wine contains 12 per cent alcohol, the number of units in the bottle is three-quarters of 12 = 9 units. If you are pouring a glass at home it is likely to be a 250 ml glass and that will contain three units not one, as you may previously have thought.

Transient ischaemic attack

A transient ischaemic attack (TIA) is often referred to as a mini stroke. By this we mean, they present in exactly the same way as a stroke (remember FAST) but the symptoms recover, sometimes within minutes but always within 24 hours. One in three people suffering a TIA will have a stroke at some point in the following year so it is important that we recognize what is happening and do all we can to reduce that risk. One in six people will have a heart attack. Reducing the risk of these events is all about doing the things that reduce your risk of a stroke generally, and taking any medication prescribed by your doctor.

How can you tell if you are going to be one of the unlucky ones?

The simple answer is you can't. None of us have a crystal ball but doctors use a scoring system to try to identify those most at risk. This is called the **ABCD score:**

- Age, being over 60 = 1 point;
- Blood pressure, greater than 140 mmHg systolic or 90 mmHg diastolic = 1 point;
- Clinical features: one-sided weakness = 2 points; speech difficulties = 1 point;

- Duration of symptoms: greater than one hour = 2 points; 10–59 minutes = 1 point;
- Diabetes, if present, 1 point.

A score of less than 4 is low risk, but if you score over 6 then there is significant risk of developing a stroke during the following week and it is important that you are reviewed by a specialist team with expertise in stroke management to minimize the risk of this happening.

3

Headaches

Almost all of us will get a headache at some point in our lives. Mostly they are a transient irritation but, for some, they can have a seriously negative impact on quality of life and, occasionally, they can be an indicator of serious disease. Interestingly, the brain itself has virtually no pain receptors. Headaches are caused by irritation of receptors in the lining of the brain (the meninges), the blood vessels, muscles, scalp, neck, sinuses, eyes and teeth.

I will discuss various forms of headache in more depth but, first, it is worth taking a few minutes to think about your headache, as your doctor will want to know various things about your headache in order to narrow down the most likely diagnosis or diagnoses. I once was taught by a professor of medicine who told me that a good doctor should have a pretty clear idea of what he or she thinks the diagnosis is simply by taking a detailed history and that examination of the patient should be to confirm those thoughts and tests to make a definite diagnosis. The longer I spend in medicine, the more I realize how true this is and it is interesting because I think patients often believe the opposite to be true and think that the more tests a doctor does, the more thorough he or she is being. You can get the most out of what is likely be, only 10 or 12 minutes with your doctor by spending some time thinking about your symptoms.

What will my GP want to know about my headaches?

- Where do you feel the headache?
- What is the nature of the headache – is it throbbing or stabbing etc.?
- How did the headache start – did it gradually build or come on suddenly?
- Does the headache keep you awake at night?
- Does the headache change during the course of the day?
- What makes the headache worse or better?
- Does the position of your head alter the headache?
- Is there a trigger for the headache, such as certain foods or stress?
- Are there associated symptoms, such as nausea or a dislike of lights (photophobia)?
- Do your eyes water or your eyelids droop?
- Has it happened before and, if so, how frequently?
- Does anyone in your family suffer with headaches?
- What pain killers have you taken, how often and do they work?
- Do you have a fever?

What will my doctor do?

Your GP will almost certainly take your blood pressure. In fact, contrary to popular belief, high blood pressure does not normally cause headaches at all but it can occasionally and your doctor will want to know your blood pressure is normal. He or she will probably look in the back of your eye, using an ophthalmoscope, for signs that could suggest raised pressure in the head and may feel your temples looking for tenderness around the temporal artery. He or she may check your temperature and look for evidence of stiffness in the neck if he or she suspects meningitis.

Will I need any tests?

The vast majority of headaches will not require any tests but if your doctor suspects temporal arteritis (see later) he or she will arrange a blood test and, if the history and examination suggest the possibility of something more serious, you may need a brain scan.

Migraine

Migraine is one of the most common causes of recurrent headache and is twice as common in women as it is in men. The headache is usually felt on one side of the head and there may be associated visual disturbance, such as flashing lights, nausea, vomiting and a dislike of bright lights (photophobia). The severity of the headache may vary from attack to attack but, typically, it is severe enough to mean that the individual cannot function during the day and may feel very tired afterwards. Migraines usually last a few hours but can last up to three days and often patients will say the pain is worse when they move their head. About one in four migraine sufferers describe what is called an **aura**. Most commonly this will be in the form of fuzzy lines in the vision of flashing lights that tend to occur a few minutes before the headache begins but can last for an hour or more.

What causes migraines?

There is often a genetic basis to migraine and, while it isn't passed on from generation to generation in a predictable way, if you have a family member who suffers with migraine you are more likely to suffer yourself. It was originally thought that migraine was caused by changes in blood vessels around the brain but scientists now believe it is caused by a wave of neuronal activity spreading across the brain followed by depressed activity spreading forwards from the back of the brain to the front.

What triggers migraine?

There are several triggers of migraine and they will vary from individual to individual. Common triggers include:

- too much or too little sleep;
- stress and recovery following a period of stress;
- hormones – migraines are common around the time of menstruation in women;
- missing meals;
- alcohol;
- over-stimulation with bright lights, strong smells or loud noise;
- foods such as chocolate, citrus fruits and cheese;
- caffeine;
- changes in climate and, especially, very cold temperatures;
- medications, such as the combined contraceptive pill, HRT and some types of sleeping tablet.

Identifying your specific triggers can be surprisingly difficult and I find getting people to keep a diary a very effective way of working out exactly what triggers their migraines. I learned this from a neurologist who had a particular interest in migraine possibly, because he was a sufferer himself. He had recurrent migraine for years and it wasn't until he took his own advice and kept a migraine diary that it became obvious where the problem lay. His migraines always occurred on a Thursday. Thursdays were his busiest day of the week. He started at his private clinic at 7 am so usually missed breakfast and got through the morning on coffee and a chocolate biscuit. There was always a Thursday lunchtime meeting where the neurologists and radiologists got together to discuss results of scans so lunch was taken on the hoof before rushing off to a busy NHS clinic. He would get home late in the evening and pour himself a large whisky. Written like this it is easy to see the pattern – and he used to joke with me that if he could have thrown in a period for good measure he was a walking textbook example of a migraine! But life is busy and it took writing things down for the pattern to become glaringly obvious.

How is migraine treated?

Unfortunately there is no cure for migraine as yet, and it may take some time for you and your doctor to work out the best treatment for you. Identifying your triggers and, where possible, avoiding them is the place to start. After that, what treatment you need will depend on the frequency and severity of your attacks. Many people will get by simply taking painkillers at the start of an attack. The earlier in an attack they are taken, the more effective they are likely to be. If vomiting is a feature of your migraine, speak to your doctor about the availability of painkillers in suppository form. If simple painkillers are not enough, your GP may prescribe a type of drug, known as **triptans**, that can be taken as a tablet, an injection or a nasal spray and which is thought to work by changing the brain activity that triggers a migraine. If taken at the first sign of a migraine, they can avert an attack. You may also be prescribed an anti-sickness medication in tablet or injection form.

Will I need to see a specialist?

If your migraines are very frequent, you may be a candidate for preventative medication so, rather than only taking pills when a migraine hits, you take medication every day to prevent them coming. This could be something called **pizotifen**, anti-epileptic medications, beta blockers, or an old-fashioned anti-depressant called **amitriptyline**.

Most migraine sufferers can be managed by their GPs and will not need hospital support, but if the treatment above is not controlling your symptoms, you may be referred to a specialist for more intensive treatment. This treatment may include:

- transcranial magnetic stimulation, which uses magnetic impulses produced by a small device held next to your head. This is generally only used for migraine with aura, and results are variable;
- botulinum toxin injections – yes, you read that right! These injections, used by many to reduce wrinkles, can be used in the scalp and neck to help prevent migraine. You will need over 30 small injections that will need to be repeated every few months;
- acupuncture.

Can I take the combined contraceptive pill if I have migraines?

It is vital you tell your doctor you suffer with migraines when you are discussing contraception. If you have migraine with aura or very severe long-lasting migraines, you shouldn't take the combined contraceptive pill as there is a very small but significant risk of stroke for these patients. If you have migraine without aura and milder symptoms, you may be able to take the combined pill but if you notice any increase in your headaches you must report this immediately to your GP.

Cluster headaches

Like migraine, cluster headaches tend to occur on one side of the head but they are generally much more painful than migraine and have been referred to as *suicidal headaches* by some because of the severity of the pain. They are called cluster headaches because this is the way they present, starting suddenly and occurring one to three times every day for weeks or sometimes months before resolving. Unlike migraine, they are more common in men, with 80 per cent of sufferers being male. They are also more common in smokers and may be associated with watering of the eyes.

What causes cluster headaches?

It is not clear what causes cluster headaches. Common triggers include:

- alcohol: cluster headache sufferers may go through phases where they can drink alcohol without adverse effects but if they drink during a cluster the symptoms are likely to flare;
- over heating: exercising in high temperatures, for example, may trigger an episode;
- strong chemical smells, such as petrol.

How are cluster headaches treated?

The treatment you require will depend on the severity of your headaches. Your doctor may prescribe strong painkillers or a triptan as used in the treatment of migraine. He or she may also prescribe high-flow oxygen, which can be used in your home. Patients who suffer with regular attacks may need a preventative medication in the form of verapamil (a blood pressure and angina treatment), lithium (usually used to treat mood disorders) or local anaesthetic injections into the back of the head.

Tension headaches

Tension headaches are very common. Unlike migraine they are usually felt on both sides of the head and patients often describe a sensation of pressure, like a band round the head or pressure on the top or front of the head. The pain is typically less severe than migraine or cluster headaches but can last for several days at a time and often builds during the course of the day.

What causes tension headaches?

We don't know what specifically causes tension headaches but they do sometimes run in families, suggesting there may be a genetic component predisposing some individuals to this type of headache. Typically, as the name implies, they tend to occur at times of emotional stress and are often linked to bad posture and physical tension in the muscles in the upper back, neck and scalp. In some people, bright lights, loud noises and extremes of temperature (hot or cold) can trigger attacks.

How can tension headaches be treated?

Managing your stress is a key factor so anything that helps relax you is good. Massage, light exercise, ideally in fresh air, and natural sunlight will help. If you spend a lot of time hunched over a computer, take a look at your posture. You should be able to sit upright with your hips and elbows at right angles, so it may be worth looking at the height of your chair and desk. Try to take breaks and walk around between jobs as much as possible. Simple painkillers from your pharmacist may be all that you need. Aspirin seems to be one of the most effective but you shouldn't take this if you are under 16, if you are asthmatic, or if you have had problems with indigestion in the past. If this isn't enough, I often use a very low dose of the old-fashioned anti-depressant amitriptyline. Patients sometimes baulk at this, but the dose we use isn't strong enough to treat depression and the drug is not addictive.

Analgesic headache

This may sound like an oxymoron but it is a very real condition. It occurs in people who take daily painkillers usually for tension or migraine-type headaches and the body becomes acclimatized to them. You then develop a type of withdrawal headache if you don't take them. This is then perceived as a further migraine or similar and the individual resorts to more pain relief. If this situation sounds familiar, have a chat with your GP who will help you gradually wean off your painkillers. It can take several weeks and a degree of faith to achieve this but it is worth doing. A similar picture can develop in patients using regular triptans and slow withdrawal works here too.

Orgasmic headache

Some people experience headaches as they orgasm. This isn't common but it is about three times as likely in men as it is in women. We don't really know why they happen but they seem to be more common in the obese, in migraine sufferers, when people are stressed and if sexual excitement is heightened. Some drugs, including marijuana, amphetamines and Viagra, also seem to be possible triggers. If you suffer and are taking any of these drugs then try stopping them; taking a more passive role in love making may also help. However, if the headaches persist, see your GP who may suggest treatment with beta blockers or calcium channel blockers. Anti-migraine therapy may also help. The good news is that for most people, even without treatment, these headaches seem to resolve in time.

Temporal arteritis

Temporal arteritis as its name implies, is inflammation – *itis* – of the artery in the temporal region, that is, the side of the forehead. We often do that in medicine – use Latin-based terms to describe a condition, which I suppose is why it was always deemed essential to have a qualification in Latin to study at medical school. It is rare in younger people, tending to occur in those over 60, and is more common in women.

What are the symptoms of temporal arteritis?

Most people develop a headache on one or both sides of the forehead. This typically builds up over a couple of days and the side of the scalp may feel tender to the touch. You may also notice that chewing food feels painful and your vision may be affected. It is common for people affected to feel like a blanket is coming down over their eyes.

Is it serious?

It can be. If left untreated, people can become blind very quickly – and I'm talking within a day or two – so if you develop a headache like this, it is vital that that you see your doctor urgently. About half of all patients with temporal arteritis develop a condition called **polymyalgia rheumatica** which causes tenderness and weakness of the muscles in the pelvic and shoulder girdles. Patients with this condition often tell me they find climbing stairs, hanging out washing or brushing their hair difficult. Women often tell me they struggle to do up their bras. If you develop any of these symptoms, don't ignore them – report them to your GP, as they may well be linked.

What will my doctor do?

If your doctor suspects temporal arteritis, he or she will arrange an urgent blood test looking for inflammation using the **erythrocyte sedimentation rate** (ESR) test or a test for **C-reactive protein** (CRP). If these tests suggest the presence of inflammation, he or she may then suggest a biopsy of the artery, which is done under local anaesthetic. If the presence of inflammation is confirmed, he or she will start you on high-dose steroids to reduce the inflammation and, hopefully, prevent any visual loss.

Are steroids safe?

Taking steroids long term is undoubtedly associated with side effects, including weight gain, diabetes, high blood pressure, thinning of the bones (**osteoporosis**) and stomach ulcers. In this instance, however, the benefits outweigh the risks and if your GP prescribes them for you, it is important that you take them straight away and continue for as long as he or she suggests. Once you have been on steroids for a while, your body becomes acclimatized to them and stops producing so much of your own natural steroid, so it can be dangerous to stop them suddenly.

How long will I need steroids for?

Your GP will monitor your progress and take regular blood tests to check on the degree of inflammation and advise you on how to gradually reduce your dose of steroids. How long you will need steroids for is an individual decision, but it may be several months.

Intracranial haemorrhage

Bleeding in the brain can cause a headache and the character of the headache alters depending on the type of bleed. The brain is covered by membranous layers, including the dura and the subarachnoid. The subarachnoid is the layer that is closer to the brain. Bleeding underneath this layer is referred to as a **subarachnoid haemorrhage**. The outer membranous layer is called the **dura**. Bleeding between this and the arachnoid is called **subdural** and bleeding outside the dura is referred to as **extradural**. I will try to explain how these are different here.

Subarachnoid haemorrhage

Some people have small dilations in blood vessels supplying the brain called **berry aneurysms**. These are like little blowouts in a tyre and cause no symptoms until they burst. When they start to leak, they cause a severe headache. People say it is like being kicked in the head. If you experience a headache like this, it is important that you seek medical attention straight away. If your doctor suspects an aneurysm, he or she will arrange an urgent CT or MRI of your head. If you have a close relative who has had a berry aneurysm, you may be at increased risk and should discuss with your GP as to whether you need a scan. People with polycystic kidneys, **coarctation** of the aorta (a birth defect where the first part of the aorta is narrowed) or an infection of the heart called **endocarditis** are also at increased risk.

What will happen if the aneurysm bursts?

Sadly, if the aneurysm bursts there is a risk you won't survive, which is why it is crucial that you seek urgent medical help at the onset of symptoms. At medical school we were always taught the rule of thirds. If a berry aneurysm bursts, a third of people make a full recovery, a third survive with some disability, and a third don't make it.

Can an aneurysm be repaired?

Yes. There are two main techniques. Either the aneurysm can be clipped, via a hole in the skull called a **craniotomy**, or an endovascular technique can be used to seal off the aneurysm. The decision on whether or not to have surgery will depend on the size of your aneurysm (the larger the aneurysm, the greater the risk of rupture), your general health and your wishes. It is vital that you are aware of the risks and possible complications before making your decision.

Subdural haemorrhage

Subdural haemorrhages are due to bleeding from a vein between the arachnoid and dural layers, and this usually follows a head injury. It doesn't need to be a particularly significant injury and the symptoms may take weeks or sometimes even months to develop so you may well not link the two events. It is more common in the elderly and in those taking medication to thin the blood. Typically, patients may develop a more low-grade headache and become a bit confused or drowsy. They may not necessarily report the symptoms themselves but if you notice these changes in an elderly relative, even if you are unaware of a particular injury, it is important that you tell their doctor.

What will the doctor do?

There are many reasons why an older person may become confused and the doctor will want to work out what is the most likely explanation. If the doctor suspects a subdural haemorrhage, he or she will arrange a CT or an MRI scan and if this confirms a bleed, the patient may need surgery to relieve the pressure on the brain.

Extradural haemorrhage

This is usually much more easy to recognize as it tends to follow a significant head injury causing a skull fracture with associated damage to an artery supplying the meninges (membranes covering the brain). The headache develops rapidly over minutes or hours and if this develops the patient will need urgent neurosurgery to remove the pressure.

How can I tell if my headache is serious?

Hopefully I have explained some of the characteristics that doctors would find concerning. People often worry that headaches are often linked to a brain tumour. Thankfully, that is not common but it is an understandable concern. The headache of raised intracranial pressure, caused by something (such as a tumour) taking up space in the brain, is generally present as soon as you wake. It is made worse by coughing, straining and even bending down and it never goes away. There may be associated visual problems. A headache like this isn't necessarily a tumour, but it mustn't be ignored and should always be reported to your GP.

Facial pain

The face has countless sensory and pain fibres, so pain in the face can be caused by a myriad of underlying conditions including dental problems, sinus disease, eye conditions and diseases of the jaw. It can also be caused by inflammation of the nerves supplying the face and one of the most common is a condition called **trigeminal neuralgia**.

What is trigeminal neuralgia?

The trigeminal nerve is responsible for supplying sensation to the face and it has several branches. In some people (usually older patients), the pain fibres appear to fire off inappropriately causing a burning sensation in the face. In younger patients this is sometimes a feature of multiple sclerosis.

How is trigeminal neuralgia treated?

Trigeminal neuralgia can be a miserable condition and ordinary pain killers generally aren't effective. Attacks can be triggered by cold wind on the face or eating hot or spicy food, so it is worth trying to avoid these. We usually use anti-convulsant medication and, very occasionally. we need to use techniques to inject the nerve or apply heat to it under anaesthetic.

4

Epilepsy

There are over 600,000 people in the UK living with epilepsy; symptoms vary from individual to individual. Electrical messages are being sent and received in different parts of our brain all the time. In epilepsy there are occasional bursts of intense electrical activity in the brain, which interrupt the normal pathways. How this manifests depends on which part of the brain is affected. This is why there are several different types of epilepsy. They are generally divided into **partial seizures**, meaning they affect only one part of the brain, or **generalized seizures.**

Partial seizures

In partial seizures, one part of the brain is affected; this may be all that happens, or they may be a warning sign that a generalized seizure is about to occur. There are two main types.

- *Simple partial seizures* These are due to electrical activity in one part of the cortex of the brain and may begin with involuntary twitching of the mouth or a single hand. This is sometimes referred to as a **Jacksonian seizure**. Activity may spread to involve jerking of one side of the body. This spread of electrical activity and visible spread, or jerking, throughout one side of the body is known as the **march** of a seizure. Sometimes there is a transient paralysis of the limbs following this kind of seizure and this is called **Todd's paralysis.** If the frontal lobes of the brain are affected you may also notice the patient's eyes looking away from the side that is jerking and the head may turn that way too.

- *Complex partial seizures* These usually begin in the temporal lobe of the brain or less commonly the frontal lobe. They are often preceded by an aura and this may come in the form of a feeling of nausea, an awareness of strange smells, visual disturbances such as objects looking a different size, or an experience of déjà vu. This is followed by a complete lack of awareness as to where the person is, which lasts a couple of minutes and which is not usually remembered by the individual after the attack. This is followed by strange movements, which vary between individuals. I have seen people making repetitive movements with their hands, walking in circles and making repetitive grimaces. This goes on for a varying amount of time and is either followed by a generalized seizure or a feeling of confusion or drowsiness.

Generalized seizures

As the name suggests these seizures reflect a more generalized electrical activity in the brain and there are several types.

- *Absence seizures (petit mal epilepsy)* These almost always start in childhood and typically you may see a child look totally vacant for a few seconds before continuing to play, as normal, with absolutely no recollection of what has just happened. They may flutter their eyelids during an attack but there are no other jerking movements. Some (but not all) children with petit mal will go on to develop grand mal epilepsy.
- *Generalized tonic-clonic seizures (grand mal epilepsy)* These are the seizures that most people will recognize as epilepsy. Some sufferers will have an aura, which warns them that a fit is about to ensue, but many won't. Typically the patient will become stiff (the tonic phase) and this is rapidly followed by the clonic phase where the patient will fall to floor and there is rhythmic jerking of the limbs. The eyes

remain open and the patient may bite their own tongue or be incontinent of urine or faeces. A fit usually only lasts a couple of minutes and during the fit the frequency of the limb jerks gradually reduces. Following this the patient will become limp and unresponsive before slowly coming round. There is then usually a period of drowsiness and confusion which may be accompanied by a headache.

Status epilepticus

Most fits will only last a few minutes, but if a fit goes on for more than 30 minutes or if there are two or more fits in rapid succession, this is referred to as **status epilepticus** and this is a medical emergency. In fact it can be fatal. The longer the fit lasts the more risky it is, as there can be permanent brain damage as a result; because of the intense muscle activity in the limbs, there can be associated muscle breakdown, which can lead to kidney failure. Surprisingly, in about half of all cases of status epilepticus, there is no previous history of seizures.

Febrile seizures

Febrile seizures are not strictly speaking epilepsy but it would be wrong of me not to mention them here, as they are common and very frightening to parents. They occur in around 1 in 20 children between the ages of 6 months and 3 years. They are, as the name suggests, associated with a fever and it seems the rate of rise of the fever is more influential than the actual temperature itself. They take a similar clinical form to a grand mal fit in that the child will become stiff and then there is jerking of the limbs. They are more likely if another member of the immediate family has suffered with febrile convulsions. Parents always worry that they herald the start of epilepsy and while there is a slight increased risk of a child with febrile convulsions going on to develop epilepsy, that risk is very small. The majority of kids suffering febrile seizures will grow out of them and not be epileptic.

What causes epilepsy?

We don't often find a particular cause for an individual's epilepsy but we do know that the following can result in epilepsy in some individuals:

- head injury
- surgery on the brain
- cerebral palsy
- brain tumours
- infection in the brain (see Chapter 10)
- stroke
- metabolic abnormalities, such as low glucose, sodium or calcium levels
- some drugs
- alcohol withdrawal
- Alzheimer's disease.

We also know that there are some triggers that are likely to provoke a fit in anyone with epilepsy and these include:

- missing doses of anti-epileptic medication
- not getting enough sleep
- flashing lights
- stress
- alcohol
- missing meals
- hormones; some women notice fits are more common around the time of their periods.

How is epilepsy diagnosed?

The diagnosis is made almost exclusively on the medical history and tests are generally done to confirm that diagnosis, so it is really important that you (or someone who has witnessed your fit as you may not remember what happened) can give a clear story to your GP. He or she will want to know the answers to the following questions.

- Was there any aura?
- What happened during the fit – what movements occurred, etc.?
- Were you confused or drowsy afterwards?
- Do you have any of the risk factors mentioned above?
- Were there any of the triggers (mentioned above) running up to the fit?
- Did you have febrile convulsions as a child?
- Does anyone else in the family suffer with epilepsy?
- What medications are you taking?
- How much alcohol do you drink?

If your GP suspects a fit, he or she will want to arrange some tests to look for a cause and confirm the diagnosis. These tests these might include:

- blood tests, to look for abnormalities of minerals or sugar that can precipitate a fit;
- a heart tracing (ECG), to rule out the possibility of an abnormal heart rhythm causing you to collapse;
- an electroencephalogram (EEG), to look at your brain waves as epileptics have characteristic changes in brain waves but we have to be careful as these can be present in non-epileptics;
- a CT or MRI scan, if a brain tumour is suspected.

Will I need treatment?

Your doctor will decide, based on your story, whether you need treatment. Often we wait and see after a single fit, as around one in five people will have no further fits and will not need long-term treatment. If, however, you have a second fit within six months of your first, then you are likely to go on to have more seizures and your doctor will recommend that you go on treatment to prevent further fits. If you have been fit free for more than two years, you may want to discuss with your doctor whether you can wean down off your medication but there is a 50:50 chance that you could have a further fit if you do.

Is there anything I can do to prevent further fits?

Since we know that there are certain lifestyle factors that can trigger a fit, it is important that you ensure that you get good nights' sleep, that you eat regularly, limit your alcohol intake, and avoid flickering lights. If you are prescribed medication, make sure that you take it as prescribed as missing doses could result in a seizure. If you are going abroad, make sure that you have enough medication to cover you while you are away.

Can I drive if I have epilepsy?

By law you must inform the Driver and Vehicle Licensing Agency (DVLA) if you have had a fit. They will tell you when you can drive again, which is usually after a year of no fits. This is also an issue if you have been fit free and considering coming down off your medication. The DVLA recommends that you don't drive while you are weaning off anti-epileptic medication and for six months after stopping. And if you were to have a further fit, then you would be asked not to drive for a further year.

Is it safe to take anti-epileptic medications during pregnancy?

In an ideal world it is better to take no medication during pregnancy, but the risk of a fit to your unborn baby is greater than medication, so you should continue your medication. If you are planning a pregnancy, talk to your doctor as some anti-epileptic medicines are safer than others and you should take an increased dose of folic acid to protect your baby from certain abnormalities.

What is sudden unexpected death in epilepsy?

If a person with known epilepsy dies suddenly without explanation it is referred to as **sudden unexpected death in epilepsy** (SUDEP). Sadly, it happens to about 1 in a 1000 people with epilepsy. We can't predict who those people will be, but we do know that there is an increased risk if you:

- have uncontrolled and frequent seizures;
- don't take medication as prescribed;
- have seizures alone or at night;
- are young and male;
- drink too much alcohol.

You can reduce your risks by attending for regular reviews with your doctor and reporting your seizure frequency so that medication can be increased as necessary. It is vital that you take medication as prescribed. If you sleep alone, you may want to consider a special alarm, which will alert others if you have a fit at night so that they can come to your assistance.

What do I do if I witness a fit?

If you witness a fit it is important to ensure that the patient is safe, so move all harmful objects from nearby. Try to cushion their head and place them on their side in the recovery position (Figure 1 overleaf). Stay with the person until the fit has finished, which should be within a couple of minutes. If the fit lasts for more than five minutes call 999. You should also call for 999 if you know this is the person's first fit, or if they seem to have injured themselves during the fit. Don't try to restrain them during the fit and don't give them anything to eat or drink until they are fully conscious.

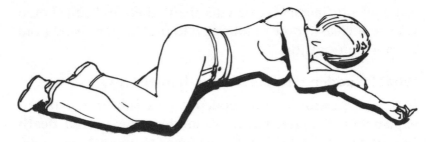

Figure 1 Recovery position

Drop attacks

These are not epilepsy as consciousness is fully preserved, but they can be mistaken for epilepsy as they cause a sudden weakness of the lower limbs, which usually means the individual collapses to the floor. They usually occur in women over 60 and are not linked to epilepsy.

Narcolepsy

This a rare disorder of sleep which causes disturbance of normal sleep patterns, meaning that the individual wakes frequently during the night and as a result may feel excessively sleepy during the day. Around a third of sufferers will have associated cataplexy. This is where there is momentary involuntary muscle weakness, often triggered by emotion. This can range from mild weakness to profound weakness, resulting in the individual falling to the floor. The attacks can last for a few minutes or up to half an hour. Narcolepsy is sometimes seen in association with Parkinson's disease or following a head injury. It is vital that sufferers try to adopt a regular sleep pattern and prescribed medication may also help.

How can I tell the difference between a fit and a faint?

At least half the population will faint at least once, most commonly as a child, during puberty or when pregnant. Faints are caused by a reflex slowing of the heart and they can be triggered by standing still for long periods, particularly in warm environments. I remember fainting in an operating theatre when I was 12. I had recently been an in-patient having had my appendix removed and was convinced I wanted to do medicine so persuaded a friend of my parents to take me into theatre to see what went on. It was a long operation and I rather unceremoniously passed out. I'm so glad it didn't put me off following my dream!

Most people experience a feeling of nausea, sweating, and or light headedness before a faint. The period of unconsciousness is very brief. There may be associated twitching of the limbs, but often the individual will lie still. When they come round they may feel a bit washed out but there is not the confusion and drowsiness as there is in a fit. If in doubt, it is important that you report any such episode to your doctor and, if possible, take someone who saw what happened with you so that they can explain the episode to your doctor.

5

Head injury

Around 700,000 people in the UK attend an Accident and Emergency department every year with a head injury and, thankfully, the vast majority of these are minor and will not require hospitalization or specific treatment. It is common to have a mild headache following such an injury. You might also feel a bit nauseous and have temporary dizziness or even blurred vision.

What is concussion?

Concussion is the term used to describe a collection of symptoms following a head injury. These include:

- ongoing headache;
- ongoing nausea and occasionally vomiting;
- dizziness or lack of co-ordination;
- confusion and irritability;
- visual disturbances, people often talk about 'seeing stars', but visual disturbances can take on many forms including blurred or double vision;
- problems concentrating;
- memory loss, this can be loss of memory of the events leading up to the head injury (**retrograde amnesia**) or loss of memory of the events occurring immediately after the injury (**anterograde amnesia**);
- slurred speech.

When is concussion serious and when should you seek medical help?

The symptoms described above are generally mild and should pass quickly but you should seek medical advice if the person who has been injured displays any of the following symptoms:

- a head injury that rendered them unconscious;
- was excessively drowsy following the event and are struggling to stay awake, especially if this is still a problem an hour or so after the event;
- a seizure;
- cannot walk properly;
- cannot read or write properly;
- a significant laceration, which may require sutures;
- bleeding from the ear;
- clear liquid leaking from the nose;
- deafness in one or both ears;
- cannot understand you or communicate.

Some people are more prone to injury following a bang on the head and these include people who:

- are over 65;
- are taking blood-thinning medication, which could predispose to a bleed in the brain;
- have had brain surgery;
- have a bleeding disorder, such as haemophilia;
- drink alcohol to excess.

It can also be very difficult to assess someone if they are drunk, as they may well exhibit many of the symptoms mentioned above – slurred speech, difficulty walking and concentrating, nausea and vomiting and so on, so if someone is drunk it is always better to be safe and get them assessed in an Accident and Emergency department.

What happens after a serious head injury?

Unlike many cells in the body, brain cells don't regenerate. Once they are destroyed they are destroyed, but the brain does have other powers of regeneration and healthy cells can take over the role of the cells that have died. Rehabilitation following a significant brain injury can take months and sometimes years as the brain has to relearn the things that you took for granted before the injury.

Patients and relatives always want to know what the future holds and that is completely understandable, but it is virtually impossible to predict outcomes in the early days. So much depends on the degree of damage and also on the personality of the individual. I have met people with horrific head injuries who have surprised everyone around them through sheer grit and determination. The support network around an individual is also very important. People who have encouragement and support from friends and relatives tend to do better than those who are isolated. What the future holds is usually clearer at about six months. I was always told that what you had achieved at a year was pretty much what you would be left with for life but, after being run over in a car accident and shattering my knee, I know that I continued to improve in year two, so I would urge anyone in rehabilitation from anything to persevere.

What should I do if I find someone unconscious?

If you come across an unconscious patient you should follow the **DRAB** criteria.

- *Danger* Check the environment for danger. If the patient is in the road, for example, make sure someone is there to stop the traffic.
- *Response* Call out to the patient to check if they respond. Shake their shoulders and see if you can get a reaction.

- *Airway* If they are not responding, lift the chin to open the airway (Figure 2).
- *Breathing* Look, listen and feel for breathing for ten seconds. If the patient is breathing, place them in the recovery position (see Figure 1 on p. 40); if the person does not appear to be breathing, you will need to breathe for them.

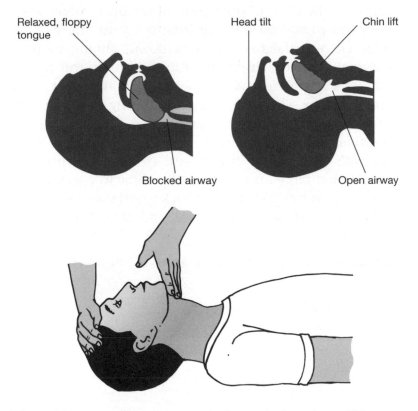

When you're unconscious, all the muscles in your body go floppy. This includes the tongue, which is a muscle. When floppy, the tongue can block the airway. The head tilt chin lift moves the tongue out of the way.

Figure 2 Head tilt chin lift to open the airway

Administering cardiopulmonary resuscitation

Administering cardiopulmonary resuscitation (CPR) involves cardiac massage to get the heart pumping, and artificially breathing for the patient, and is sometimes referred to as **giving the kiss of life:**

- *Chest compressions* Place the heel of your hand on the centre of the chest in the region of the breast bone. Place your other hand on top and interlock your fingers. Lock your elbows straight and press down, aiming to press down about five centimetres. You need to do this repeatedly at a rate of around 100 beats per minute and do 30 compressions. This is the same as pressing to the rhythm of 'Nelly the Elephant' or 'Staying Alive'.
- *Breathing* Lift the chin with two fingers and pinch the patient's nose. Cover the mouth completely with your mouth and blow in, watching the chest to check that it rises. Repeat this and then go back to chest compressions. Another 30 chest compressions and then back to two rescue breaths.

You will need to repeat this cycle until medical help arrives.

6
Brain tumours

Brain tumours are, thankfully, not very common. About half of all brain tumours are actually due to secondary spread from a cancer elsewhere in the body. We call these **metastases** and they can come from cancer in the lung, breast, stomach, bowel, skin, prostate, thyroid or kidneys. Of the remaining brain tumours, 35 per cent will be cancerous and 15 per cent will be benign. Each year, about 9,400 people are diagnosed with a brain tumour in the UK. There are many different types and they can affect all ages: 400 children are diagnosed with a brain tumour each year.

Who gets brain tumours?

Although a brain tumour can strike at any age, they are more common as we get older. Other risk factors include:

- exposure to radiation, which increases the risk of both benign and cancerous brain tumours;
- having had a previous cancer – adults who had cancer in childhood or who previously had leukaemia or lymphoma are at increased risk;
- family history, as some brain tumours have a genetic component or may be linked to inherited conditions such as neurofibromatosis or Turner's syndrome;
- late stage HIV infection;
- obesity, which increases the risk of benign meningioma;
- smoking, which may increase the risk of developing some brain tumours.

Does living by a power line or using a mobile phone increase risk?

There has been lots of talk about both of these issues but as yet no proof that either is associated with an increased risk of developing a brain tumour. One theory is that, if there is any increased risk of using a mobile phone, it is more likely to be a problem in the developing brain – in other words to children. This is by no means proven and I am happy to let my kids use mobile phones as they wish, but I do ask them not to charge them by their beds overnight.

How would I know if I had a brain tumour?

The symptoms of a brain tumour are due to pressure effects within the skull. The skull is a bony box with no room for expansion, so as a tumour grows it puts pressure on the brain. In the early days you may have no symptoms at all but as the tumour grows it causes symptoms; exactly which symptoms you experience will depend on where in the brain the tumour is growing. Symptoms can include:

- headaches
- nausea
- drowsiness
- fits
- problems with your vision.

It is important to remember that many of these symptoms are very common and, in the vast majority of people, will be due to something far less serious. We all get headaches, for example, but the headache from a brain tumour is usually quite severe. Patients wake up with the pain in the morning and anything that raises pressure in the head will make the headache worse. If you have a bad headache that persists, and is worse on coughing, sneezing or bending, you should get it checked out.

More specific symptoms are related to the position of the tumour.

- *Frontal lobe* The frontal lobes are linked to our personality so a tumour here may mean you behave differently: you may lack enthusiasm for things, become irritable or aggressive. Some patients become disinhibited or may find it difficult to concentrate. Tumours here can also cause weakness in the face or limbs, difficulty walking and talking and a loss of sense of smell.
- *Temporal lobe* The temporal lobe is where we store memory and process sound, so a tumour here may mean you find it difficult to find the correct word for things, you may have short term memory loss or have feelings of déjà vu. Sometimes people even hear sounds or voices in their head which are not actually there.
- *Parietal lobe* The parietal lobe is where we process the words people say to us and where we process the sensation of touch, so a tumour here may mean you have problems speaking or understanding what is being said to you. You may not be able to feel parts of your body.
- *Occipital lobe* The occipital lobe is responsible for sight. A tumour here may cause sight problems or even blindness.
- *Cerebellum* The cerebellum is responsible for co-ordination. A tumour here will cause problems with balance and fine motor skills like writing.
- *Brainstem* The brainstem controls vital functions that we perform without conscious thought, such as heart beat, breathing and swallowing. A tumour here may mean you have difficulty swallowing.
- *Pituitary gland* The pituitary gland sits right in the middle of the brain and controls the production of hormones, including fertility and growth hormones. A tumour here may cause period problems in women, infertility and enlarged hands, feet and jaw. Tumours here can also cause

visual problems because of a pressure effect on the optic nerve as it runs next to the gland.

- *Acoustic neuroma* The nerve between the ear and brain is called the **acoustic nerve**. If a tumour develops here it causes one-sided hearing loss.

How are brain tumours diagnosed?

If your doctor suspects a brain tumour from your story, he or she will want to examine you and, if your doctor is still concerned, he or she will arrange a CT or an MRI scan of your brain to look for a tumour. You may also need more detailed tests following the scan, such as PET or SPECT scans, angiograms or neuroendoscopy (see Chapter 1).

What are the different types of brain tumour?

There are 130 different types of brain tumour. Some are benign and others cancerous or malignant. Tumours are graded by how quickly they are likely to grow. A pathologist looks at the tumour under a microscope and grades the tumour 1–4. Grades 1 and 2 are considered low grade, and 3 and 4 as high grade. The tumours are named according to the tissue in which they grew.

Gliomas are the most common form of primary brain tumour and there are three main types:

- **astrocytoma**, which account for a third of all brain tumours. They grow in the cells supporting the nerve cells called the **astrocytes**.
- **oligodendroglioma**, which are rare. They originate in the myelin which is the protective layer of nerve fibres that helps nerve conduction.
- **ependymomas**, which are also rare. These tumours originate in the cells lining the ventricles and spinal cord.

Other forms of brain tumour are:

- **meningiomas**, which account for a quarter of all brain tumours. They are more common in women and older people. They grow in the meninges lining the brain and are generally considered benign, but they do sometimes recur after being removed.
- **haemangioblastomas**, which develop in the blood vessel cells and tend to be very slow growing.
- **acoustic neuromas** start in the nerve between the ear and the brain. They are generally benign.
- **craniopharyngiomas** are exceptionally rare and occur at the base of the brain.

How are brain tumours treated?

How your brain tumour is treated will depend on the type of tumour, its size, its grade and where it is positioned. You may be offered any combination of surgery, radiotherapy and chemotherapy. The decision will be made by you and your team, which is likely to include neurosurgeons, neurologists, oncologists and radiologists.

Can I drive if I have a brain tumour?

Your doctor will tell you if you are obliged to tell the DVLA. Not all tumours need to be reported. An acoustic neuroma does not need to be reported, for example, unless it has caused dizziness. If you have had a fit as a result of your tumour, you will not be allowed to drive again until you have been fit free for a year. In most instances you will not be able to drive while you are being treated for a brain tumour and for a variable period afterwards. This is usually six to twelve months, depending on the type of tumour and the treatment you have had.

7

Memory and dementia

Human memory is immensely complex and precious. Most weeks, I see someone concerned that maybe they are losing their memory. I often describe memory as a suitcase. We are born with an empty suitcase and throughout our lives we put things in that case. When it is relatively empty, it is easy to put in new things but, as it gets full, there is less and less space. Eventually, it is full up to bursting and every time we try to put something new in, something else has to be displaced. In fact, it is not that simple because when we lose our memory, it is the memory for recent events (the things we have only just placed into the suitcase) that goes. If you spend some time talking to anyone with dementia, you find that they may have no idea what they had for lunch an hour ago, or indeed whether they even had lunch, or what day it is, but they may be able to remember their wedding day or wartime experiences in minute detail. It is normal to become forgetful with age, and I try to reassure people it is completely normal to forget where you put the car keys. What is not normal is to forget what they are for.

Which part of the brain controls memory?

There is no one part of the brain that is responsible for memory. We have all heard people talk about the fact that once you have learned, you never forget how to ride a bike. I once heard a doctor give a lecture on exactly this to illustrate how complex memory is. In order to ride a bike you need to be able remember how you physically balance on it and move the pedals, you need to remember the route to take to get you from A to B and you need to remember the highway code to make sure you are safe on the roads and to look out for other road users. These memories are all very different and involve different parts of the brain.

When we remember events we need to retrieve the information from our memory bank and this is done in one of two ways. Short-term memory is retrieved sequentially. So if someone reads you a limerick and then asks you to repeat the third line, you will read through the limerick in your head, or out loud, in order to retrieve the information; or if you go into the kitchen to get something and can't remember what you were looking for, when you go back to where you came from that often triggers your memory. Long-term memory, however, is stored and retrieved by association, which is why you may find yourself feeling emotional at a particular song before you have consciously remembered the significance of that song.

What causes memory loss?

There are many things that cause loss of memory and sometimes it can be as simple as you weren't really concentrating when the information went in. So if you are reading a newspaper when someone asks you to phone the window cleaner, you may well not remember. That's not because you are losing your mind, it's because you weren't really listening at the time and it wasn't a priority to you. If the same day you were reading the same newspaper you had been offered tickets to see your favourite band play live, you would remember because you would have shifted your focus of attention. Other factors that influence our memory include:

- age, we all get more forgetful as we get older not because of dementia, but because our suitcases are full;
- mental health problems, stress, anxiety and depression can all affect our ability to concentrate and may affect memory;

- head injury, minor head injuries can cause short term memory problems but more significant injuries may cause longer term issues;
- stroke;
- brain tumour;
- alcohol, drinking excessively one night may mean you can't remember what happened the following morning, and long-term alcoholics are also at risk of longer-term memory problems;
- hypothyroidism, an underactive thyroid can leave you feeling lethargic and excessively sleepy, which will affect your memory;
- infections, a chest or urine infection may cause confusion and memory problems particularly in the elderly;
- drugs, any drug that has a sedating side effect can impair your ability to remember. If you think your memory is going downhill since starting a new medication, discuss it with your GP. Don't ever be tempted to stop a prescribed drug without talking to your doctor, but do have the conversation as there may well be an alternative that you find more acceptable.

What can I do to boost my memory?

Your brain is like anything else – if you don't use it, you risk losing it! So, stretch your brain, keep it active. It doesn't matter whether that means doing quizzes and crosswords, reading or learning poetry, if your mind is active it will be more likely to stay that way. If you know you are getting forgetful, write things down, set alarms for yourself and try to set up a routine so that you know where you put things.

I am often asked whether *Ginkgo biloba* helps memory. It is thought to work by improving blood flow to the brain.

Research studies don't all agree, but it may be worth a try; it doesn't seem to work as a preventative for dementia but it may help in boosting memory. As with any herbal remedy, I have two simple rules. The first is always tell your doctor if you are taking a herbal remedy as they may interfere with some conventional medicines. Ginkgo, for example, has blood thinning properties. The other is to opt for a preparation that has a patient information leaflet in the packaging. Herbal remedies are not as tightly regulated as medicines, but some manufacturers volunteer to have their products regulated and these products will have a leaflet inside, so you know what you are getting.

What will my doctor do if he or she suspects a memory problem?

Your GP will want to know what it is that you are worrying about specifically, and you may find it useful to take a close friend or relative with you to explain the potential problem. If you are at all concerned that you have a memory issue, then do write down what you want to say. We all forget things in the pressure of an appointment but if you are genuinely forgetting things, it is much more likely to be an issue. Your doctor may want to do some tests to rule out some of the conditions I have mentioned above and will also do a mini mental state examination (Table 1 overleaf).

What is dementia?

Dementia is the most serious form of memory loss and the one that people always worry about. In the UK, there are more than 850,000 people living with dementia. It is progressive, although very variable in the way it progresses.

There are three main types – Alzheimer's disease, multi-infarct dementia and Lewy body dementia, which I will discuss in detail below. Dementia can also be caused by other medical conditions such as alcohol abuse, syphilis and various vitamin deficiencies. Your GP will check for these.

Table 1 Mini mental state examination

		Maximum score
Orientation	What is the year/season/date/day/month?	5
	Where are we – country/county/town/hospital/floor?	5
Registration	Name 3 objects: 1 second to say each. Ask the patient all 3 after you have said them. Give 1 point for each correct answer. Then repeat until he/she learns all 3. Count trials and record.	3
Attention and calculation	Serial 7s. 1 point for each correct answer. Stop after 5 answers. Alternatively, spell 'world' backwards.	5
Recall	Ask for the 3 objects repeated above. Give 1 point for each correct answer.	3
Language	Name a pencil and a watch.	2
	Repeat the following: 'No ifs, ands or buts'.	1
	Follow a 3-stage command: 'Take a paper in your hand, fold it in half and put it on the floor.'	3
	Read and obey the following: CLOSE YOUR EYES.	1
	Write a sentence.	1
	Copy the design shown.	1

Who gets dementia?

Dementia is most common in the elderly but it can affect anyone and I have met very young, previously mentally agile, people whose lives have been wrecked by the condition. The things that increase your risk of dementia include:

- family history
- low IQ and learning disabilities
- head injury
- Parkinson's disease (see Chapter 8)
- mental health problems, severe depression and schizophrenia
- cardiovascular risk factors, including high blood pressure, high cholesterol, diabetes, obesity, smoking and lack of exercise.

The three main types of dementia

Alzheimer's disease This is named after the doctor that first described the condition. It is a gradually progressive loss of memory and brain function and is the most common form of dementia. It is thought that proteins build up in the brain and prevent the normal electrical messages getting through. Ultimately, this leads to death of nerve cells and loss of brain matter. There is also a shortage of the chemicals that are used to pass messages between nerves in the brain. In the early stages of the disease, individuals may just seem forgetful. They may forget a special birthday or what you were just talking about, but as the disease progresses they may find it difficult to follow the conversation in the first place. They may forget to turn the oven off, or that they have left the front door wide open. This can be frustrating and that can manifest itself as outbursts of aggression. Ultimately, the person becomes unable to care for themselves and needs 24-hour care and supervision. I am often asked how long this process will take and, sadly, it is impossible to tell. Some people decline very gradually over many years and, unfortunately, other people experience a much more aggressive deterioration. One study suggests that on average it takes around seven years from diagnosis (if you are under 70) before you become totally dependent.

Multi-infarct (vascular) dementia This is dementia that is caused by mini strokes in the brain and, clinically, it differs from Alzheimer's in that rather than a gradual decline in mental function, you are more likely to see stepwise decline with each mini stroke.

Lewy body dementia This is named after the abnormal protein deposits that are found in this form of dementia. It may present in the same way as Alzheimer's or multi-infarct dementia but if the deposits are formed in the brainstem, patients may also develop symptoms similar to Parkinson's disease (see Chapter 8).

What can I do to reduce my risk of developing dementia?

Anything you can do to keep your brain active will help. Do puzzles and games, try to stimulate your mind with conversation and reading. You should also do everything you can to lower your risk by reducing your cardiovascular risk. There are several changes to lifestyle that can influence your blood pressure and cholesterol level and could prevent you developing dementia. This is essentially the same advice that was given in Chapter 2 as a way to reduce the chances of suffering a stroke.

- *Smoking* If you are a smoker you should stop now. Your GP and pharmacist will be able to help you. Most surgeries now run smoking cessation clinics where you will be able to discuss which methods appeal most to you. Some people use nicotine replacement, others may choose pills to help with the cravings and some may swap to electronic vaping devices.

- *Weight* If you are overweight, you should aim to lose weight gradually – one to two pounds a week – until you are a healthy BMI, which is between 18.5 and 25. You can calculate your BMI by dividing your weight in kilos by the square of your height in metres. So, if I am 1.63 m tall and weigh 52 kg, my BMI is:

$$BMI = 52/ (1.63 \times 1.63) = 19.5$$

- *Diet* It is important that you aim to have a healthy well-balanced diet. Watch your fat intake – only a third of your total calories should be fat and you should limit your intake of trans fats and saturated fats to a third of your total fat intake. This means limiting your intake of butter, cheese, pastries, cakes and biscuits. It will also mean getting into the habit of checking food labels for fat content. This may seem laborious at first but you will soon get to know which foods you should avoid. You should eat at least five portions of fruit and vegetables a day. A portion is a single apple, orange or banana; two plums or apricots; 30 g of dried fruit; two broccoli spears; one medium tomato or seven cherry tomatoes; three heaped tablespoons of beans; or 150 ml of unsweetened fruit juice. However, because fruit juice has less fibre you can only count one glass into your five a day. And potatoes don't count as vegetables in this context. Watch your sugar intake too, and beware 'low fat' options – always check the labels as 'low fat' often means 'high sugar'. You should also eat two portions of oily fish each week; this includes mackerel, sardines, kippers, salmon, pilchards, herring or fresh tuna.
- *Salt* We have got used to a high salt diet in the western world. You should limit your daily intake to 6 g. Start by not adding salt to your food. At first this will taste bland

but human taste buds adapt very quickly and by using herbs and spices you will soon wonder how you ever managed to eat such salty food! When you start looking at the hidden salt in processed foods you will be shocked by the amounts.

- *Exercise* You should aim to do half an hour of exercise at least five times a week. It doesn't matter what you do. It doesn't have to be in a fancy gym but you should choose something you enjoy doing so that you will stick with it and, even better, if you can exercise with a friend then you will encourage each other when your willpower is weak. So whether is a brisk walk, cycling, jogging, swimming or dancing, you need to be exercising at a level that makes you out of breath. If you are gasping for breath then you should ease back a bit but if you can chat away easily while you are doing your exercise then you are kidding yourself and you need to up your game!

- *Alcohol* Drinking to excess can lead to an increase in blood pressure, so make sure you stick to recommended limits of alcohol – that is 14 units per week for women and 21 for men – and try to have at least two dry days per week. A unit is actually probably a lot less than you think. The simple way to calculate your alcohol intake is by looking at the percentage alcohol in the drink you are drinking. The percentage alcohol shows you the number of units in a litre of that drink; so, for wine, a 75 cl bottle is three-quarters of a litre (75 cl = 750 ml; 1 litre = 1000 ml), so if the wine contains 12 per cent alcohol, the number of units in the bottle is three-quarters of 12 = 9 units. If you are pouring a glass at home it is likely to be a 250 ml glass and that will contain three units not one, as you may previously have thought.

Can medication help with dementia?

Your GP may prescribe medication to control high blood pressure or cholesterol if this is an issue for you and, if multi-infarct dementia is suspected, you may be advised to take a low dose of aspirin. Dementia patients are often also prescribed an anti-depressant, as depression is a common feature. There are also specific drugs used to treat the symptoms of dementia. Sadly, there is no cure as yet for dementia but your doctor may suggest you try the drugs to treat the symptoms, and the decision on whether you should have any of these drugs will be made on an individual basis:

- *acetylcholinesterase inhibitors* Acetylcholine is the chemical that is transmitted between nerves and it is reduced in patients with dementia. There are strict guidelines on the use of acetylcholinesterase inhibitors; they must be started by a specialist and progress must be closely monitored. It is only used for as long as it is deemed to be making a difference. They work in about half of patients who try them.
- *memantine* This drug reduces the chemical glutamate and seems to slow down damage to the brain cells, and therefore progression of dementia, in some patients.

Is there anything else that can be done?

I think of this as the four Rs, and it is really advice for dealing with friends or relatives with dementia.

- Routine – If a person with dementia has a regular routine and things are always put in the same place, it is much easier for them to remember.
- Repetition – Try to be patient with someone suffering dementia. It can be frustrating for all concerned but being prepared to repeat things means they are more likely to remember.
- Reminders – Leave notes, set alarms and text or ring to

remind your nearest and dearest about appointments, medications and meals.
- Reminiscence – Encourage dementia sufferers to talk about the past. You may be pleasantly surprised by what they can remember and they will enjoy the experience.

Can I drive with dementia?

If a formal diagnosis of dementia is made you are obliged to tell the DVLA. You may be allowed to continue to drive for quite some time, but you may be asked to repeat your driving test if there are concerns and your GP may be asked to provide a medical report. Some people with dementia find manoeuvring a car more difficult as they may develop problems with spatial awareness, and if you have got to the stage where you are forgetting where you go then you may decide that driving is no longer for you anyway.

What is transient global amnesia?

Transient global amnesia is a sudden, complete, yet – thankfully – temporary loss of memory. Patients can't remember where they are, what they are doing and repeat the same questions over and over again as they simply don't remember your answer. They remember who they are and their friends and relatives. An attack is short lived (usually less than 24 hours) with a gradual return of memory. Episodes can be triggered by stress, physical exertion, immersion in hot or cold water, sexual intercourse, medical procedures or a relatively minor head injury. Transient global amnesia is more common in migraine sufferers and tends not to occur in people under the age of 50. As it is so short lived and rarely recurs, there is no specific treatment other than reassurance and supervision during the episode.

Creutzfeldt-Jakob disease

Creutzfeldt-Jakob disease (CJD) is a rare and fatal condition caused by an infectious protein called a **prion**. It affects fewer than two people in every million each year in the UK. There are four types of CJD:

- **sporadic** CJD is the most common form, thought to be caused by a spontaneous change in protein in the brain;
- **variant** CJD is the form that you will have read about in the newspapers as it thought to be caused by eating meat from a cow infected with **bovine spongiform encephalopathy (BSE; mad cow disease)**, which is a similar prion disease;
- **familial or inherited** CJD is exceptionally rare, affecting one in nine million people;
- **iatrogenic** CJD is where the infection is spread through medical or surgical treatment. It used to be a problem with growth hormone treatment as the growth hormone used to be taken from the pituitary gland of dead people who may have had CJD. Now that we know the risks, iatrogenic CJD is almost unheard of.

CJD is a horrid disease that causes progressive decline in intellectual function, visual problems and blindness, changes in personality, uncontrolled jerky movements, speech difficulties and loss of mobility. At the moment there is no cure for this disease.

8

Parkinson's disease and movement disorders

Parkinson's disease

There are 127,000 people in the UK living with Parkinson's disease. It is rare under the age of 50. It is caused by a lack of a chemical called **dopamine**, which is involved in transmitting neurological signals from the brain and, specifically, from an area in the brain called the **substantia nigra**. A lack of dopamine means the signals coming from the brain to the muscles are slowed down. We don't really know what causes it, but rural living, drinking well water and exposure to pesticides have all been put forward as possible risk factors. Some drugs can cause a Parkinsonian picture as a side effect. It is thought that there is also a genetic component in some cases.

How would I know if I had Parkinson's disease?

Parkinson's disease develops slowly and in the early stages it may not be obvious, but it is a progressive disease. The main features are slowness, rigidity and tremor.

- Slow movements, also called **bradykinesia**, are a classic feature of Parkinson's patients. Patients find it difficult to get out of a chair or out of bed and get going, and they tend to shuffle when they walk. The facial muscles don't move as actively, meaning they look blank and expressionless.
- Rigidity occurs because the muscles become stiff and, rather than moving smoothly they tend to jerk and move in a slightly robotic way that doctors call **cogwheel rigidity**.

- Tremor, the tremor of Parkinson's is described as a 'pill rolling tremor'. It most commonly affects the hands and is most pronounced at rest, becoming less obvious when the hands are busy doing something.

Other features include small handwriting, difficulty swallowing, slow monotone speech, poor balance and fatigue. Sadly, as the disease progresses, patients often become incontinent, have difficulties sleeping and are more likely to have problems with anxiety and depression. They may also notice changes in their sense of smell and may see and hear things that are not there.

How is Parkinson's disease diagnosed?

There isn't a specific test to diagnose Parkinson's. I can't take a sample of blood or put you through a scanner to confirm the diagnosis. Instead we make the diagnosis on the clinical picture. It can be difficult in the early stages but as the disease progresses the slowness, tremor and rigidity become more apparent and the diagnosis is clearer.

How is Parkinson's disease treated?

Unfortunately, there is no cure for Parkinson's so treatment is aimed at improving the symptoms and this is done by using drugs designed to boost levels of dopamine in the brain. These include:

- **levodopa**, which is the precursor to dopamine. The body converts levodopa to dopamine. Levodopa is given in combination with another drug to stop this conversion occurring in the bloodstream and to ensure that it occurs in the brain where the dopamine is needed. Unfortunately, over time levodopa works less well and doses need to be increased. At higher doses, side effects are common and these include uncontrollable jerky movements, which patients often find exhausting. Some patients have a gel infusion of levodopa placed directly into the small intestine.

- **dopamine agonists** mimic the effects of dopamine and are sometimes given in combination with levodopa.
- **monoamine oxidase inhibitors** block an enzyme that breaks down dopamine and so help to enhance the levels of dopamine in the brain.
- **catechol-O-methyltransferase inhibitors** work by preventing the breakdown of levodopa.

As the disease progresses, you are likely to also have input from physiotherapists, occupational therapists, who may be able to advise on adaptations to your home to make day to day life easier, and speech therapists, if there are problems with speech or swallowing. Work is also being done on deep brain stimulation. This is where electrodes are tunnelled under the skin and implanted deep in the brain and electrical impulses are then sent into these parts of the brain to improve symptoms. There is also work being done looking into transplanting dopamine-rich tissue from embryos into the brains of Parkinson's sufferers.

Can I drive if I have Parkinson's?

If you are diagnosed with Parkinson's, you must tell the DVLA and your insurance company. You may need to have a medical assessment but you will be able to drive until the disease progresses to the point that you would not be able to react safely.

Other movement disorders

Huntingdon's disease

Huntingdon's disease is usually an inherited condition where there is progressive damage to the brain resulting in changes in mood and personality and uncontrolled fidgeting and jerky movements. In about 3 out of a 100 cases there is no genetic link but in the majority of cases there is, and if one of your parents has the disease you have a 50:50 chance of developing it. The diagnosis is made on the clinical picture and confirmed by genetic testing. Sadly, there is no cure.

Essential tremor

This is an inherited condition. Just like Huntingdon's disease, if one of your parents has the condition you have a 50:50 chance of developing it too. It tends to start quite early in life and affect mainly the hands, but can also affect the head and neck. The tremor gets worse under periods of stress and, unlike Parkinson's disease, gets worse when the hands are in use, as when holding a cup or a pen. It may not need treatment but beta blockers and some anti-epileptic medication may help.

Tics

Tics are common. They are repetitive movements usually affecting the face and neck, although they can affect any part of the body. Perhaps the most well known form of tic is Tourette's syndrome, which is characterized by multiple motor tics and at least one vocal tic. It is three times as common in boys as it is in girls. We don't know as yet why it happens but it is often associated with **attention deficit hyperactivity disorder** (ADHD) or **obsessive compulsive disorder** (OCD).

Dystonias

Dystonias are conditions where there is uncontrolled muscle spasm and contraction. We don't know exactly why they develop but it is thought to be due to a problem in the part of the brain, called the **basal ganglia**, which controls movement. They can occur as a result of Parkinson's disease, after a stroke or following brain injury. They can be treated with muscle relaxing drugs and botulinum toxin injections. In severe cases, surgery to divide the nerve ending causing the spasm can be tried.

9

Multiple sclerosis

Multiple sclerosis (MS) affects about 80,000 people in the UK. It is two to three times more common in women than in men and symptoms tend to occur first between the ages of 20 and 40. It is more common in Caucasians and occurs more frequently the further from the equator you live; even in the UK, MS is more common in Scotland than it is in the south of England. MS seems to be an immune-mediated condition that attacks the nervous system. Nerve fibres have a protective layer, called the **myelin sheath**, which helps messages travel quickly between the brain and the rest of the body. In MS, the myelin is damaged, meaning that these messages are slowed down, distorted or blocked completely.

What causes MS?

We are yet to identify a specific cause for MS, but we do know that a mixture of genetic and environmental factors seem to play a role.

Genetics There is not a specific gene that is linked to MS, but it seems multiple genes interact to increase the risk, which is why there is a very small increased risk of developing MS if you have a first degree relative with the condition. Most of the genes that have been linked to MS relate to immune system function.

Environmental factors There is some evidence that a viral infection could trigger MS in the susceptible, especially infection with the Epstein Barr virus, which is the virus that causes glandular fever. Low vitamin D levels have also been implicated, which would explain the increased prevalence in regions with less daylight that are far away from the equator. Smoking may also increase the risk and this may be because smoking affects our immune system.

How would I know if I had MS?

The symptoms of MS are hugely varied. About a quarter of sufferers will present with visual problems, commonly pain around the eye and loss of vision in one eye, but any nerve can be affected. The typical picture is one of sporadic neurological symptoms, which sometimes improve. These symptoms can include the following.

- *Visual disturbances* These can take any form from complete loss of vision to blurred or double vision.
- *Sensory symptoms* Patients sometimes describe a strange sensation like water is trickling down their skin. You may notice numbness or pins and needles anywhere on your body.
- *Motor symptoms* You may find that you are clumsy, or your co-ordination has deteriorated and you are unsteady on your feet. You may have muscle spasms, which can be quite painful.
- *Urinary symptoms* You may develop urinary urgency and frequency, and this may mean you wet yourself if you can't get to a toilet quickly as the bladder contracts uncontrollably.
- *Pain* This may be linked to muscle spasms but may also occur with no obvious explanation. This is called **neuropathic pain**.
- *Fatigue* This is common and may seem out of proportion to other physical symptoms but can be very debilitating.
- *Temperature sensitivity* An unusual feature is a temporary worsening of symptoms following exercise or a hot bath when body temperature has risen.
- *Electric shock sensations* Some patients experience a sensation

like an electric shock down the arms when they look down and put their chin on their chest.
- *Depression* This, understandably, is a common feature of MS.

How is MS diagnosed?

There is no one diagnostic test for MS, but if your doctor suspects the diagnosis, he or she may arrange any of the following:

- MRI scan, to look for the plaques of demyelination;
- lumbar puncture, to look for changes in the proteins in the cerebrospinal fluid;
- visual evoked potentials, to test how quickly your brain responds to visual stimuli as in MS the responses are slowed.

Lumbar punctures and visual evoked potentials used to be common tests for MS, but now that MRI scans are more readily available they are done less frequently.

What are the different forms of MS?

There are three different forms of MS.

Relapsing-remitting MS This is by far the most common form, accounting for about 90 per cent of cases. The relapses describe the onset of a new neurological symptom, which may last anything from a few days to several weeks before subsiding, which is called a remission. The frequency and severity of the relapses is variable. Typically, this remitting and relapsing pattern may last several years and often there is full recovery between episodes but eventually, after several years, there seems to be progression to permanent damage.

Secondary progressive MS This is considered late stage MS and 75 per cent of people with the relapsing-remitting form of MS will eventually develop this form of MS, resulting in permanent nerve damage and varying degrees of disability.

Primary progressive MS About 10 per cent of MS sufferers will develop this form of MS and develop slowly progressive symptoms from the outset.

How is MS treated?

Sadly, we do not yet have a cure for MS so treatment is aimed at easing symptoms. Along with medication, you may need input from physiotherapists, speech therapists, occupational therapists, psychologists and, if you need adaptations to your home, social services. We know that MS is an immune-mediated disease, so many of the drugs used are aiming to modulate the immune system and these include **interferon** and drugs called **monoclonal antibodies**. Most of these have to be given in injection form. They are specialist drugs, which are started by hospital neurologists not your GP. High-dose steroids are also helpful, given by mouth or directly into the vein to reduce inflammation during a relapse. Your GP may also give you painkillers, drugs to reduce muscle spasms and drugs to help control your bladder.

Is cannabis legal to use in MS?

The use of street cannabis remains illegal but there is a cannabis extract available on prescription. There is still a lot of debate as to whether there is any proof of the benefits of cannabis in treating MS, and NICE advise against its use on the NHS.

What is the outlook following a diagnosis of MS?

MS is a very different disease in different people so it is difficult to predict how you will do. There is no doubt in my mind that a positive attitude improves the prognosis and many people with MS continue to work and live independently for many years. The fewer your relapses and the better your recovery between attacks, the better your outlook.

10

Infections of the nervous system

Meningitis

Meningitis is inflammation – *itis* – of the membranes surrounding the brain and spinal cord – the meninges. It can be caused by:

- viruses, including the viruses that cause mumps, chickenpox, influenza, HIV and glandular fever;
- bacteria, including Neisseria, streptococci, listeria, haemophilus, *E. Coli* and the bacteria that cause TB and syphilis;
- fungi, including candida (the fungus that causes thrush).

Viral meningitis

Viral meningitis is the most common form of meningitis and is generally less serious than bacterial meningitis. It usually resolves within 10 days. The headache may persist for several months, but there are rarely more serious consequences.

Bacterial meningitis

This is less common but much more serious as it is often accompanied by blood poisoning (**septicaemia**). Interestingly, some of the bacteria that cause meningitis can live harmlessly in the nasal cavity of about 25 per cent of the population. Close contact (kissing, coughing or sneezing) can pass the bacteria to others. We don't know why, but it can then take over the immune system in vulnerable individuals and cause meningitis. The very young (pre-school children) and teenagers seem to be most at risk.

Fungal meningitis

This is much less common and occurs in people who are known to have a weakened immune system, such as people on chemotherapy or who have end-stage HIV infection.

What are the symptoms of meningitis?

In the early stages a child may just look unwell, be off their food, may feel sick and develop a fever. This is followed by developing cold hands and feet, which look pale or dusky and mottled. The child may be irritable or drowsy. Older children may complain of a headache, a dislike of bright lights or stiff neck. The classic meningitis rash doesn't always appear but, if it does, it starts as red or purple spots that look like blood blisters. These often develop rapidly and spread, sometimes coalescing to form patches. If you notice a rash like this in an unwell child, you should perform the glass test. Simply roll a glass over the rash. If the spots do not blanch, this is likely to be the rash of meningitis and it is a medical emergency. You need an ambulance immediately. The sooner antibiotics are given, the better the outlook. Unfortunately, if treatment is delayed, a previously healthy child can be dead within hours. However, if antibiotics are started soon enough, most people make a full recovery. Some, however, will have long-term problems following bacterial meningitis and these include brain damage, deafness, epilepsy, kidney failure, bad scarring or even the need to amputate a badly affected limb.

How can meningitis be prevented?

You only have to meet one bereaved family or one child badly affected by the aftermath of meningitis to believe in the value of vaccination. We are very lucky here in the UK to have a pretty comprehensive childhood vaccination pro-gramme. In years gone by, mumps was a relatively common cause of viral meningitis and one that we see much less frequently now because of the MMR vaccine. Thousands of

column inches have been written about the possible association between the vaccine and autism. A lot of research work
has been done since the possibility was first proposed and
there is no proof of any link. Suffice it to say, all three of
my children had both doses of the MMR and I would do the
same today. Children are vaccinated against haemophilus
(Hib), group C meningococcus and pneumococcus and there
are also plans to vaccinate young children against group B
meningococcus in the near future.

Should I be worried if I have been in contact with someone with meningitis?

Meningitis is a notifiable disease, which means that doctors
are obliged to report all cases. Close contacts of anyone diagnosed with meningitis will be offered a course of antibiotics
to protect them. By close contacts, we mean those people
who share a house with the patient or people who have been
kissing the patient in the week before the illness developed.

Encephalitis

Encephalitis is inflammation of the brain. It is usually caused
by viruses, the most common being the herpes simplex virus,
which is the virus that causes cold sores and genital herpes.
Other common culprits include the viruses that cause chickenpox, mumps, measles and flu. It can affect anyone, but
the very young and the very old seem to be most at risk.
Unlike meningitis, it is very rare for bacteria or fungi to cause
encephalitis.

How would I know I had encephalitis?

The symptoms can be vague in the early stages. You may just
feel generally unwell with a fever, aching limbs, nausea, vomiting and a headache. This is followed by worsening of the
headache, confusion and drowsiness. You may have a stiff
neck, weak legs and a dislike of bright lights (photophobia).

You may go on to have a seizure and lose consciousness. If you recognize these signs in anyone, call for urgent medical attention.

How is encephalitis diagnosed?

If your doctor suspects encephalitis, he or she will order an urgent scan of your brain. This could be a CT scan or an MRI scan depending on availability. You may also have a lumbar puncture to collect fluid from around your spinal cord, which will then be analysed in the laboratory. You may also have an electroencephalogram (EEG), which shows characteristic changes in the brainwaves if encephalitis is present.

How is encephalitis treated?

If doctors suspect encephalitis, they will probably start anti-viral treatment even before test results are available because time is of the essence. The sooner effective treatment is started, the better the outlook. If treatment is delayed, encephalitis can be fatal or leave individuals with significant disability such as deafness, blindness, speech problems, mobility problems, difficulties with memory and concentration, and personality changes.

Can encephalitis be prevented?

Vaccination against chickenpox, influenza, measles, mumps and rubella helps to prevent encephalitis caused by these viruses.

Shingles

Most viral infections are cleared from the body fairly quickly after infection. The chickenpox virus (**herpes zoster**) is different. Following an episode of chickenpox, the virus crawls back up the nerve endings and goes to sleep. It may stay asleep, but sometimes it reactivates and crawls back down the nerve to cause shingles. The rash of shingles looks like chickenpox, so it starts with small blisters, which then ulcerate and crust over. In chickenpox, the rash is all over the body. In shingles it is just in the band of skin supplied by the affected nerve and it doesn't cross the midline of the body, as the left and right side of our bodies are supplied by different nerves. It can take three or four weeks for the crusting to heal. Some people notice a burning or tingling sensation in the skin for a few days before the rash develops.

Why does the virus reactivate?

Shingles reactivates when our immune system is low. It can happen when we are chronically stressed and run down or, less commonly, it can be a sign that there is a more significant underlying problem with the immune system. Ultraviolet light also seems to be a trigger. The classic scenario, which I often see in surgery, is the person who is totally run down and finally books a sunshine holiday to take a break and is then knocked down with shingles.

Is shingles infectious?

The vesicles (rash) on the skin are teeming with chickenpox virus, so if you were in contact with someone who had not had chickenpox or who had a weakened immune system, for example from chemotherapy, they could catch chickenpox from you. You can't catch shingles from shingles.

Are there any long-term problems with shingles?

About one in ten people have ongoing pain at the site of the rash many months after the rash has healed. If the trigeminal nerve is involved, ulcers may develop on the cornea of the eye causing scarring and visual problems. If the facial nerve is involved, one side of your face may droop. This is called a **Bell's palsy**.

How is shingles treated?

The sooner antiviral treatment is started, the better the outlook. If you recognize the tingling sensation in your skin, it is worth starting the medication at the onset, before the rash has even developed. You can reduce your risk of shingles by trying to manage your stress levels and using a high sun protection factor sunscreen. If you develop **post-herpetic neuralgia**, you will need prescription medication from your GP as normal painkillers are not usually enough to relieve the pain. If you have lesions around the eye, you must see your doctor immediately and, similarly, if you notice a facial droop, which will need steroid treatment. If you are 70, 78 or 79 and registered with an NHS GP, you will be offered a vaccine against herpes zoster. Vaccination against herpes zoster reduces the incidence of shingles by 50 per cent.

Syphilis

You may wonder why on earth I am talking about syphilis in a book on brain health. After all, it's a sexually transmitted infection, isn't it? Yes it is, but it is an unusual infection in that it has different phases.

- The primary phase produces painless sores on the genitals or around the mouth which last two to six weeks.
- The secondary phase, which occurs after the sores have healed, produces a rash that develops over the body (often the palms and soles) and a sore throat.
- The tertiary phase can cause blindness, deafness, dementia or a stroke.

Tertiary syphilis can occur many years after the other two phases and the effects that it can have on the brain is the reason for the inclusion of syphilis in this chapter. It is rare in the UK, but worth a mention as it is serious. Tertiary syphilis needs a long course of antibiotics, often given into a vein in the arm. Sadly, this won't reverse any existing damage but it will prevent further neurological complications developing.

11

Peripheral nerve diseases

Motor neurone disease

There are several types of motor neurone disease (MND). The most common is also referred to as **amyotrophic lateral sclerosis** and that is what I will concentrate on here. We don't know why it happens, and we don't know why the disease should attack only some nerves. Motor neurone disease, as its name implies, only affects the motor nerves. There are no sensory symptoms at all. There is no loss of intellect, no problems with memory and no difficulties hearing or seeing. In fact, the person is fully aware throughout the disease. It is just the muscles that become weak. Think of Stephen Hawking – a man with a phenomenal brain but whose muscles have completely let him down.

What are the symptoms of MND?

Motor neurone disease is a slowly progressive disease. In the early stages you may just feel you are being a bit clumsy. You may drop things more easily or trip more often. You may find it difficult to walk upstairs or get out of a low chair. You may notice a change in your singing voice or feel that your speech is a bit slurred. You may also notice that sometimes your muscles flicker uncontrollably. The symptoms progress such that eventually you are unable to walk, you may not be able to talk and you may have difficulty eating and swallowing.

How is motor neurone disease diagnosed?

If your doctor suspects motor neurone disease from your story, he or she will want to examine you. Your doctor will take some time assessing the strength of your muscles by asking you to resist movement. He or she will look at your muscles to see if they have started to waste away and also look for **fasciculations**, which are tiny quivering, flickering, movements in the muscle. Sometimes these can be provoked by tapping the muscle. There is no one specific test to diagnose the condition, but nerve conduction tests to check the speed at which electrical impulses pass through your muscles and a special scan to measure the activity of nerves between your brain and spinal cord are used to help confirm the diagnosis.

How is motor neurone disease treated?

Sadly, there is no cure for motor neurone disease but there is a drug, called **riluzole**, which slows the progression of the disease by a few months. Not surprisingly many patients become depressed and need anti-depressant medication. Other treatments are introduced to deal with the symptoms as they progress. Some patients will need feeding tubes, electronic gadgets to help them communicate and help with breathing in the later stages of the disease. People always want to know how long they will survive and it's a difficult one to answer as the disease can be very variable but, as a rough guide, sadly 70 per cent will die within 5 years of the onset of symptoms and only 1 per cent will still be alive at 10 years.

Guillain-Barré syndrome

Guillain-Barré syndrome is an unusual condition where the nerves throughout the body become damaged following an infection. It is more common in women than men and can occur a few weeks after infection with a virus or bacteria. Common triggers include food poisoning, glandular fever and some forms of pneumonia. It is thought that when the body makes antibodies to fight the infection, then in some people those antibodies attack their own nerves.

What are the symptoms of Guillain-Barré syndrome?

Symptoms usually start within three weeks of an infection and they tend to start peripherally. So, weakness and tingling or numbness in the hands and feet may be the first sign. The legs are affected more than the arms and about half of all sufferers will also experience pain. The symptoms can spread up the body over the next month and in severe cases the muscles of the chest wall become involved, which makes breathing difficult. If the muscles of the mouth and gullet are involved, then swallowing is affected.

How is Guillain-Barré diagnosed?

If your doctor suspects Guillain-Barré from your story, he or she will arrange for a lumbar puncture looking for high levels of protein and white cells. He or she may also do some nerve conduction tests.

How is Guillain-Barré treated?

You will be looked after in hospital in the early days as symptoms can progress rapidly and you will need to be monitored to check that you can breathe and swallow normally. You may be given an injection of immunoglobulin to boost your immune system. Most people will make a full recovery in six to twelve months.

Peripheral neuropathy

This a term used to describe the condition where the peripheral nerves are damaged. It can affect any nerve but most commonly first affects the extremities.

What causes peripheral neuropathy?

There are many possible causes and they include:

- diabetes
- excessive alcohol, or other causes of liver disease

- kidney disease
- cancer
- vitamin deficiencies
- physical injury
- underactive thyroid
- toxicity from arsenic, lead or mercury
- medications.

What are the symptoms of peripheral neuropathy?

The symptoms will depend on which nerves are affected.

- *Sensory nerves* Damage in these nerves may cause numbness, tingling or a burning sensation, and difficulties with balance.
- *Motor nerves* Damage here may cause muscle twitching and wasting and weakness.
- *Autonomic nerves* Damage to these nerves may cause constipation or diarrhoea, problems with sweating, low blood pressure, palpitations and urinary or sexual problems.

One nerve may be involved, in which case it is called a **mononeuropathy**. If multiple nerves are involved, this is called a **polyneuropathy**.

How is peripheral neuropathy treated?

The most important thing is to identify and treat the underlying cause so your doctor may need to do several tests to work out what is causing your problems. Symptoms may be eased with steroid treatment and drugs to suppress the immune system. Immunoglobulin injections are also helpful. The pain of neuropathy doesn't usually respond to normal painkillers and your doctor may try old-fashioned antidepressants in low doses or anti-epileptic medication to get the pain under control. We also sometimes used a cream made from the extract of chilli peppers.

12

Sleep

When we sleep, we sleep in cycles described as rapid eye movement (REM) sleep and non-REM sleep. As the name implies, your eyes are closed during REM sleep, but they are very active moving quickly in different directions. During non-REM sleep the eyes remain still. REM sleep is a lighter sleep, during which we dream. Non-REM sleep is a deeper sleep. If people sleepwalk or sleeptalk, this occurs in non-REM sleep, which is why people remember dreams but usually have no recollection of sleepwalking or sleeptalking. I have met people who have gone downstairs and made a sandwich, but have no memory of it whatsoever! An old wives' tale says that you mustn't wake someone if they are sleepwalking, as it will give them a heart attack. Like all old wives' tales there is a grain of truth in this. If you wake someone who is sleepwalking, you take them from their deepest sleep to awake in a very quick time frame, which can be distressing to the individual but not fatal.

Normal sleep patterns

In normal healthy sleeping, there are three phases of non-REM sleep.

- *Stage 1* Your eyes are closed but you are easily roused. This lasts up to 10 minutes.
- *Stage 2* Light sleep where you heart rate slows down and your core body temperature drops.
- *Stages 3 and 4* Deep (or slow wave) sleep where it is more difficult to rouse you. It is during this stage that your body

repairs, you grow and your immune system strengthens. Your blood pressure falls and your breathing slows.

After about 90 minutes of non-REM sleep, you have your first episode of REM sleep. The first period of REM sleep lasts for about ten minutes. You then go back into non-REM sleep before further episodes of REM sleep, and this cycle repeats itself four or five times during the night with each episode of REM sleep lasting a little longer. The final period of REM sleep lasts about an hour. REM sleep accounts for about a quarter of total sleep time in adults and more than half of an infant's sleep. Sleep patterns are regulated by chemicals in the brain and an internal body clock that responds to daylight and means we feel awake during the day and sleepy at night.

How much sleep do we need?

Most adults need seven or eight hours of sleep a night, although there is huge variation between individuals and the simplest way to gauge whether or not you are getting enough sleep is on how you feel when you wake. If you wake feeling refreshed and ready to tackle the day, you have had enough sleep. If you wake feeling exhausted, you have not had enough sleep. This isn't a problem on an occasional basis but chronic lack of sleep will affect your mental agility and physical health. Babies need much more sleep, because they are developing rapidly, and so need nearer 17 hours of sleep per day.

Why do we need sleep?

Sleep allows the body to rest and replenish energy stores and allows the brain to process memories, so it is important for learning. It also strengthens the immune system. Chronic sleep deprivation has been linked to depression and learning problems, but also to increased susceptibility to infection. It can also contribute to high blood pressure and can alter the way we metabolise sugar so can increase the risk of diabetes and obesity.

How can I improve my sleep pattern?

If you are having difficulty sleeping, there are a number of things you should try.

- Avoid any caffeine after 6 p.m. and remember that tea also contains caffeine. Opt for a herbal tea, such as chamomile.
- Take regular exercise but avoid exercising late at night as this will increase adrenalin levels and make you feel more alert.
- Avoid sleeping during the day. It can be difficult when you feel so tired but it will disrupt your usual sleep pattern.
- Don't rely on alcohol. It may help you to get off to sleep but it disrupts the normal sleep cycles meaning you wake feeling less refreshed.
- Check the temperature of your bedroom as being too hot or too cold will affect your sleep.
- Avoid eating big meals immediately before bedtime.
- Try to deal with any worries or plans before going to bed. If you have things on your mind, keep a pen and paper by your bed. If you wake worrying about things you can write them down and then they are out of your mental in-tray and can be dealt with in the morning.
- If you are not asleep within 20 minutes, get up and go and read or watch something soothing until you feel tired. Beds should be for sleeping and sex so try not to read in bed if you are someone who has difficulty getting off to sleep.

Some of my patients have found the herbal remedy valerian helpful. If you are still struggling then speak to your doctor. Sleeping tablets are very effective if there is an acute problem such as bereavement, separation or work stress, but they are highly addictive and shouldn't be used long term (that is, for more than two weeks).

Sleep apnoea

Sleep apnoea is a condition where the airways become blocked and people stop breathing in their sleep. If you sleep on your own, you may not be aware there is a problem other than you may feel excessively sleepy during the day, or feel moody and irritable. If you sleep with someone else, they may notice that you snore loudly and then have periods where you seem to stop breathing altogether. Sleep apnoea is more common in men than it is in women and tends to occur in people who are overweight. The diagnosis is made by monitoring your sleep overnight in a sleep laboratory where your breathing and brainwaves can be observed. Mild cases can usually be managed with weight loss, but in severe cases, you may need to wear a mask at night which is attached to a continuous positive airways pressure (CPAP) machine to keep your airways open at night.

Index